Healthy Cities

Healthy Cities

EDITED BY
John Ashton

OPEN UNIVERSITY PRESS
Milton Keynes · Philadelphia

Open University Press
Celtic Court
22 Ballmoor
Buckingham
MK18 1XW

and
1900 Frost Road, Suite 101
Bristol, PA 19007, USA

First Published 1992
Reprinted 1992

British Library Cataloguing-in-Publication Data

Healthy cities.
  I. Ashton, John
  307.76

  ISBN 0-335-09477-5
  ISBN 0-335-09476-7 pbk

Library of Congress Cataloging-in-Publication Data

Healthy Cities/edited by John Ashton.
      p.   cm.
  Includes index.
  ISBN 0-335-09477-5 (hb)   ISBN 0-335-09476-7 (pb)
  1. Urban health.   I. Ashton, John, 1947–   .
  RA566.7.H43   1991
  362.1'998—dc20   91-21246
                                                  CIP

Typeset by Best-set Typesetter Limited, Hong Kong
Printed in Great Britain by
St Edmundsbury Press Ltd, Bury St Edmunds, Suffolk.

This book is dedicated to the urban poor and to all those committed to working for social justice and urban ecological sanity. It is in memory of Duncan, the other early pioneers and the founders of the Health of Towns Association

Contents

Contributors

Antoinette Ackermann, Australian Capital Territories Community Health Association, Canberra

Carlos Alvarez-Dardet, Professor of Public Health, University of Alicante

John Ashton, Senior Lecturer and Head of Department of Public Health, University of Liverpool and Visiting Professor at the Valencian School of Public Health

Frances Baum, Director, Southern Community Health Research Unit

Knud Bragh-Matzon, Healthy Cities Co-ordinator, Horsens, Denmark

Concha Colomer, Senior Lecturer in Health Promotion, Valencian School of Public Health; Associate Professor, Department of Community Health, University of Alicante

Janine Cosijn, Health Promotion Officer, Eindhoven Healthy Cities Project

Jaume Costa, Healthy Cities Co-ordinator, Barcelona

M. Dobranovi, Social Worker, Ministry of Health and Social Welfare, Zagreb

Len Duhl, Professor of Public Health and City Planning, University of California, Berkeley

S. Ferint, Center for Mental Health, Zagreb

Beverly C. Flynn, Project Co-ordinator, Healthy Cities Indiana

Peter Flynn, Corporate Policy and Information Manager, Liverpool City Council

Lela F. Folkers, Acting Chief, Health Promotion Section, Department of Health Services, Sacramento, California

Geoffrey Green, Healthy Cities Co-ordinator, Liverpool

Joseph M. Hafey, Executive Director, Western Consortium for Public Health, Berkeley, California

Trevor Hancock, Public Health Consultant, Ontario

Trudy Harpham, Head of Urban Health Programme, London School of Hygiene and Tropical Medicine

Ricardo Garcia Herrera, Public Health Director, Gobierno Vasco, Spain
Flemming Holm, Horsens Healthy Cities Project, Denmark
Lewis Kaplan, Inaugural National Co-ordinator for Healthy Cities Australia
S. Lang, Project Co-ordinator, City Assembly of Zagreb
Genaro Astray Mochales, Public Health Officer, Gobierno Vasco, Spain
S. Sogoric, Assistant Professor of Social Medicine, Healthy Cities Team, Zagreb
Elizabeth Rasmusson, Consultant, Pan American Health Organization
Marilyn Rice, Regional Adviser in Health Education, Pan American Health Organization
Melinda Rider, Associate Project Co-ordinator, Healthy Cities Indiana
Ann Skewes, Human Services Co-ordinator, South Australian Urban Land Trust
Ingvar Svensson, Head of Public Health Department, City Office, Gothenburg, Sweden
Hoane Kataka Takarangi, Curator of History, Manawatu Museum, Palmerston North, New Zealand
Janet Takarangi, Quality Management Consultant, Palmerston North, New Zealand
Gavin Thoms, Consultant in Public Health Medicine, Sheffield Health Authority
Joan M. Twiss, Project Director, Healthy Cities Project, Western Consortium for Public Health, Sacramento, California
Jan van der Kamp, Healthy Cities Co-ordinator, Eindhoven
Judy Whyte, Healthy Cities Co-ordinator, Canberra

Foreword

Why are networks of cities being developed in all parts of the world? City Networks may be formed to achieve a variety of goals, for example the Metropolis City Network was formed to promote urban development and housing, environmental protection, urban transport, the urban economy, urban management, and health; the UN Economic and Social Commission for Asia and the Pacific developed its CITYNET network to promote better urban management.

City Networks can provide the following benefits:

1 Sharing of information between members.
2 Sharing of scarce resources to solve joint problems, for example developing effective urban management strategies.
3 Joint development of standards or codes of good urban policies and management practices; the existence of such standards then has the effect of exerting pressure on all members of the network to adopt them, for no member wishes to become a bad example.
4 City Networks have the potential to provide a force to influence national policies and norms to promote healthy urban development. This force can for example promote the decentralization of urban management functions and urban development decision-making from the national government level to the municipal government level, that is essential to allow local participation in urban development.

Since 1986, WHO Regional Office for Europe has been utilizing a deliberate strategy of city networking, the purpose of which is to put health on the social and political agenda of cities in Europe. The project seeks to bring together political and community leaders, local citizens, community organizations, professional associations and national and international agencies in a collaborative, intersectoral and community-based effort to achieve health for all at the local level.

Networks and coalitions for health have been established within cities, between cities nationally and internationally, and between cities and key national and international agencies.

The success of this strategy can be judged by the fact that what was originally envisaged as a project of limited appeal involving four to six cities has mushroomed to involve thirty Project Cities in Europe, seventeen National Networks (several outside Europe) involving hundreds of cities, towns and villages, and a wide range of national and international agencies. What started as a project is fast becoming a movement! Indeed all six of WHO's regional offices, which service virtually all countries in the world, are developing Healthy City networking approaches as a major strategy in their urban health development efforts.

It is most fitting that John Ashton has edited this important book, for he has been an active and vital presence in the Healthy Cities Project from its inception and has continued to support the process as it develops in the Middle East, Asia and Africa. The intelligence, energy and commitment he brings to the project will be apparent to all readers.

Greg Goldstein
Division of Environmental Health
WHO Geneva

Preface and acknowledgements

Success has 100 parents, failure is an orphan.

When a small group of us sat around a table in Copenhagen in January 1986, we had no way of knowing that the Healthy Cities Project, which we were proposing, would acquire such an active life. The original idea was that between four and six cities would develop local action plans for health promotion based on Health for All principles (WHO 1981). Within a short time, the project had all but been eclipsed by a world-wide movement of city-based public health initiatives. This really was an idea whose time had come . . . again. Ideas like this have no one author – they are a manifestation of serendipity, of people being tuned in to the moods and ideas of their times and giving them a push in the right direction. In one sense the Healthy Cities Project was a new initiative, in another it was the Health of Towns Association of Exeter 1844 reborn.

Many people have invested enormous amounts of energy in this idea since it was first mooted. The group of people with whom I sat around the table on a snowy January day in Copenhagen consisted of:

Keith Barnard
Len Duhl
Trevor Hancock
Ilona Kickbusch
Constantino Sakellarides
Michael Suess
Jill Turner
Harry Vertio

They were soon to be joined by Eric Giroult, Tjeerd Deelstra, Bob Tanner, Gunter Conrad, Marie Bistrup and Ron Draper, with the committed support of the secretarial staff, especially Bente Drachmann, Sue Line Irmov, Tina Peralta and Linda Petersen. More recently Marilyn Rice (in PAHO, Washington, DC), Ashley Files, Jo Hafey, Joan Twiss, Beverly Flynn, Melinda Rider and John Parr have been active in promoting the initiative in the United States and the Americas, and Fran Baum, Antoinette Ackermann, Judy Whyte, Richard Hicks, Hero Weston, Val Brown, Lewis Kaplan, Louise Croot and Janet Takarangi in Australia and New Zealand. Dr M.I. Sheikh and Q. Khosh Chasm in Alexandria and Greg Goldstein, Dr Tarimo and Dr Tabibzadeh in Geneva have been responsible for the most recent developments in the Middle East, Asia and the Pacific. In 1991, the technical discussions of the World Health Organization chaired by the British Chief Medical Officer, Sir Donald Acheson, focussed on health in urban areas, marking a profound shift of emphasis and indicating that the health crisis of the cities is now being recognized.

Within a short time, many other people have become involved and it would be invidious to try and identify them all. All of the authors in this volume have made major contributions to the New Public Health and this book is dedicated to all my co-workers. I would also like to thank Celia Vishnick and Sonia McKeown for their uncomplaining dedication to a somewhat uncontrolled task.

The Health of Towns Association achieved the objective of Public Health legislation within four years. The objectives of Healthy Cities are wider and more ambitious. They are part of a movement whose focus is Social Justice in Health and Ecological Sanity for the Planet. This will take longer than four years to achieve, but we believe that we have made a good start.

John Ashton
Liverpool

Reference

WHO (World Health Organisation) (1981) *Global Strategy for Health for All by the Year 2000*, Geneva: WHO.

City 2000 by Adrian Henri

In this city
filled with the sound of alarm-bells
police sirens howl
like animals mating,
vagrants huddle together
in cardboard cities;
in a damp bed-sit
a girl dreams visions of Patmos,
cool white spaces,
the dusk gleam of an icon,
THE NIGHT
written in dripping white
on a railway wall.

swarming city,
city full of dreams . . .

In this city
the sound of the bulldozer is banished from the
land,
swingeing custodial sentences imposed
on anyone designing a building
finished in shuttered concrete.

Carparks burst into flower
narcissi, blue-flags, lilies-of-the-valley
pushing up through the tarmac,
the streets heaped with yellow marigolds,
All planning decisions are referred to
the postman Ferdinand Cheval
Charles Rennie Mackintosh
and
Antoni Gaudi
(all speaking though a medium).

This city
no longer an embarrassment,
the too-much-loved-mother
at the School Speech Day,
lipstick blurred,
smelling of gin-and-lime.

As the sun rises over
this city,

your morning face on the pillow
through strands of dark brown hair,
the river lying back open to the day,
the lace curtains of terrace-houses
sing like schoolchildren.

This city
is your mother,
and your lover.

She is your first thought,
and your last.

She is your future,
and your past.

We are most grateful to Adrian Henri for permission to use his poem which is also reproduced
by permission of Rogers, Coleridge & White Limited.

Vol 3 No 3.

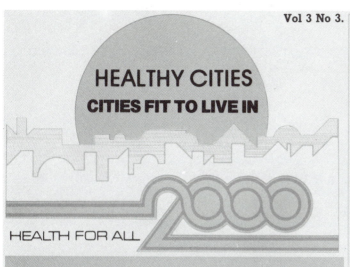

HEALTHY CITIES
CITIES FIT TO LIVE IN

HEALTH FOR ALL **2000**

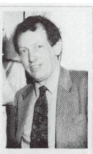

An information exchange newspaper produced by the Healthy Cities Centre, supported by the Division of Strengthening Health Services, WHO, Geneva.

Advanced Health Centres point the way to reorientating Urban Health Systems

report by John Ashton

The experiences of cities from nine countries in developing advanced or 'reference' urban health centres, was the focal point of a recent meeting of the World Health Organisation.

The meeting was held against a background of the rapidly emerging concern for the precarious state of health of people living in cities throughout the world. This concern has 3 elements.

● The accelerating pace of urbanisation such that the infrastructure cannot keep up with the urban growth.

● The demographic and health transitions with ageing populations and the increasing importance of non-infectious and chronic disease including accidents and trauma. In addition AIDS is creating an immense threat to urban health systems in some countries

● The cost crisis of medical care systems which are based on hospital

Liverpool schoolchildren have been on an unusual 'tour' of Europe — See page six for more details.

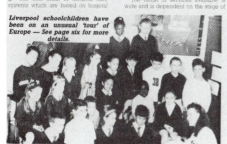

and inpatient care.

Since 1978, the implementation of new patterns of health care based on the eight activities of primary health care identified in the Alma Ata declaration has been carried out with varying levels of success.

There exists a dynamic situation where new technologies and procedures taken together with clinical and social management protocols have made outpatient ambulatory and day centre care a practicable, high quality and potentially cost saving alternative to inpatient care.

Various countries have now developed examples of integrated community health and medical care centres to provide those services most appropriately delivered at the local level to tackle the prevention, cure and rehabilitation of common local conditions (endemic disease)

The range of services available is wide and is dependent on the stage of

development of the country and of local health services. The approach seems to be relevant to rural as well as to urban areas and has the potential for significantly changing both the style and content of hospital provision in urban areas. The Geneva meeting in May 1991 heard that typically the range of services provided includes :

— Health promotion, health education, preventive medicine and primary health care

— Maternal and child health including family planning and services relating to reproductive health

— Environmental health services

— General medical care

— Community-based nursing and social care

— Out-patient services including day surgery and treatment, urgent care of minor accidents and emergency treatment, diagnostic procedures and rehabilitation

— Short stay inpatient care

Reports of extended primary health care initiatives which included some or all of these elements were given from Alma Ata, Bombay, Cali, Jakarta, Karachi, Manila, Mexico City and Dakar as well as an account of the development of day surgery care in the United Kingdom.

In Cali, there is now 20 years experience of a university and community partnership approach to the provision of enhanced primary health care which incorporates ambulatory surgery, normal deliveries emergency care, rehabilitation, sterilization, neonatal care, complex diagnostics and outpatient care.

● Continued on page 2.

HEALTHY CITIES:
reorientating urban health systems is the key

The World Health Assembly technical discussions were a watershed in placing urban health firmly on the agenda. The General assembly of WHO accepted resolutions supporting the extension of Healthy City type initiatives on a global basis. However, what is becoming clear is that the reorientation of urban health systems is a prerequisite to achieving urban Health for All. A recent WHO consultation in Geneva heard evidence about just how effective systems can be when they adopt a Health for All approach. The idea of the reference health centre in an urban setting is gathering momentum, and examples of these are reported in this issue from as far apart as Alma Ata, Bombay, Cali, Jakarta, Karachi, Mexico City, and Dakar.

Typically, the extended range of services in such a centre includes health promotion, preventive medicine, maternal and child health, environmental health general medical care, community based nursing and social care, outpatient services, and short stay in patient care.

Here are practical examples of how the medical sector can make a major contribution to the development of Healthy Cities.

The front cover of a recent United Kingdom Healthy Cities Newsletter.

1

The origins of Healthy Cities

John Ashton

A historical context

On 11 December 1844 the Health of Towns Association was formed at a public meeting at Exeter Town Hall. Finer (1952) describes it as an 'avowed propagandist body...of capital importance'. At this first meeting, it was stated that the Association was to be formed with the purpose of sharing information gained from recent inquiries made into the terrible living conditions of much of the population. The aim was to work for changes in the law which would improve the public health.

This initiative and others like it were part of a response to the threat posed to Public Health by industrialization and rapid urbanization. Throughout Europe the poor were living in appalling, insanitary conditions, crowding into urban slums and vulnerable to epidemic infectious disease. Governments seemed reluctant to introduce reforms; the Health of Towns Association was a body which could play an important part in pressurizing the government into reform.

Following the first meeting in Exeter, Lewis (1952) describes how branches were quickly formed in Edinburgh, Liverpool, Manchester, York, Halifax, Derby, Bath, Rugby, Marlborough, Walsall, Plymouth and Worcester. The local branches worked by disseminating facts and figures drawn from the official reports, by organizing public lectures on the subject, by reporting on the sanitary problems of their district and by organizing public meetings to petition Parliament. Their focus was upon the deliberations of the Health of Towns Commission, which had been set up by the government in 1843 and had been led by Edwin Chadwick (1965) into producing detailed reports on the poor conditions existing in the cities. It was from these deliberations that what came to be known as 'the Sanitary idea' emerged – the notion that overcrowding, inadequate sanitation and the absence of safe water and food created the conditions under which epidemics could thrive. The response was seen to lie in housing standards and hygiene regulations, paved streets and publicly funded water and sewerage systems.

A flavour of the activities of one branch of the Health of Towns Association can be had from an account of the first Liverpool meeting which was convened by the Mayor in April 1845. A feature in the *Liverpool Mercury* (25 April 1845) describes the attendance at this first meeting as being 'not large but highly respectable', including leading members of the council, and both Protestant and Catholic clergymen, in addition to Dr William Henry Duncan (later to become the country's first city Medical Officer of Health). The *Mercury* describes those present as 'gentlemen of all sects in religion and all parties in politics'. This meeting passed unanimous resolutions defining the sanitary objective to be aimed at and called for legislative action. The duty of the Association should be to collect funds, to supply information and to furnish those details which must be the basis of all legislation. The meeting set up a local committee which published the monthly *Liverpool Health of Towns Advocate* for nearly two years – 1,500 copies of the first issue being distributed free of charge.

According to White (1951), the working classes were not well represented in the Liverpool Association although they were the worst sufferers from insanitary conditions. However, White feels that the Association did a good job of bringing an appalling situation to people's attention. Until this time, it seems that many citizens were under the impression that Liverpool was one of the healthiest towns in the country. The evidence that was provided shocked people into calling for action to be taken by appealing to a combination of civic pride, humanitarianism and enlightened self-interest – for the evidence showed that the poor were not the only sufferers from the insanitary conditions; the gentry in Liverpool had worse mortality rates than the gentry in Leeds and London.

The growth of the Liverpool Health of Towns Association led to other bodies becoming concerned about public health. One example was the Liverpool Guardian Society for the Protection of Trade, which conducted an inquiry into the city's water supply in 1845. White (1951) describes how they concluded that the Liverpool water supply was not only miserably inadequate, but also almost the most expensive in the country. There were suspicions expressed that the supply was deliberately restricted to keep up monopoly profits and it was suggested that it would be better if the water supply were to be unified under a public authority.

The work of the Health of Towns Association in pressing for the application of the sanitary idea and its insertion into public policy-making had a dramatic effect on public health in Britain in a comparatively short space of time. The various campaigning groups and branches were effective on the national, as well as on the local, stage and in 1848 the Public Health Act of Parliament unified the legislation and organizational arrangements for Public Health. Once this legislation had been effected, and with the passing of the threat of cholera, Lewis states that the popular enthusiasm for sanitary reform rapidly subsided. The campaigners left behind them an approach and a menu of measures which had flowed from the sanitary idea which can be summarized as follows:

1 The legitimacy of working locally.
2 Resourcefulness and pragmatism.
3 Humanitarianism and a strong moral tone.
4 The recognition of the need for special skills and qualifications.
5 Appropriate research and inquiry.
6 The need to focus on positive health.
7 The value of producing reports on the state of health of the population.
8 Populism.
9 Health advocacy.
10 The need for persistence and working with trends.
11 The need for organization.
12 The recognition that public health needed to be the responsibility of a democratically accountable body.

In addition it is clear that they established what we would now call (in WHO jargon) an intersectoral coalition to work for public health. The lessons which are to be learned from this period of British Public Health are well described in the collected writings of Sidney Chave (1987).

From the sanitary idea to the new public health

The sanitary idea with its environmental focus continued to exert a central influence in public policy in developed countries until towards the end of the nineteenth century, when the germ theory of disease paved the way for immunization and vaccination which introduced a shift of emphasis from environmental action towards personal prevention. In turn this era was superseded by the therapeutic era, dating from the 1930s with the advent of insulin and the sulphonamide drugs. Until that time it has been argued by McKeown (1976) that there was little of proven therapeutic efficacy available. Since the 1930s and until the early 1970s, public policy on health in Britain and in many other countries was dominated by a treatment orientation and an implicit assumption that magic bullets could be provided by the pharmaceutical industry for all conditions.

By the early 1970s the therapeutic era was increasingly being challenged. Most countries were experiencing a crisis in health care costs, not least those developing countries which had been misled into adopting the new Western fashion of large hospitals and cadres of expensively trained professionals; the first of these siphoned off the bulk of the health care budget leaving little for the rural areas or for primary care, the second undermined the traditional practitioners without replacing them as new professionals proved reluctant to work outside the fashionable areas of the large towns. From this experience, the twin concepts of Primary Health Care and an emphasis on Community Development began to emerge.

In the United Kingdom, McKeown's statistical analysis which demonstrated that most of the decline in infectious disease mortality in England and Wales between 1840 and 1970 preceded effective therapeutic intervention, provided a powerful rationale for a revived interest in public health and preventive medicine. McKeown (1976) concluded that, in order of importance, the major contributions to improvements in health in England and Wales had been

1 limitation of family size (a behavioural change)
2 increase in food supplies
3 a healthier physical environment (environmental influences)
4 specific preventive and therapeutic measures.

McKeown also made the point that disease tends to occur in populations when species stray too far from the environmental conditions under which they evolved.

McKeown's work provides a constant reference point in what has come to be known as the New Public Health – an approach which draws crucially from the environmental, personal preventive and therapeutic eras and seeks a synthesis. Its focus is on public policy as well as on individual behaviour and lifestyle and increasingly it is being seen in an ecological context which has a focus on holistic health. One of the key events in the development of this new momentum for public health was the publication in 1974 of the Lalonde Report – *A New Perspective on the Health of Canadians* – in Canada. This report was in essence a restatement of the tradition of public health reports leading to policy which went back to Chadwick, but which, ironically, was about to be abandoned as one of the consequences of local government reorganization in the United Kingdom. The kind of community diagnosis which the Canadian report represents has since been taken up around the world and at different levels of population aggregation; with the WHO Healthy Cities Project it has helped to stimulate the revival of city health reports.

Since the Lalonde Report was published (1974), shape has been given to the new public health movement by a series of initiatives from the World Health Organization, starting with the Alma Ata declaration on Primary Health Care in 1977 and culminating in the Healthy Cities Project in 1986. The central elements of these initiatives are a focus on the condition of the poor and less advantaged, the need to reorientate medical services and health systems, away from hospital care and towards primary health care and the importance of public involvement and of partnership between the public, private and voluntary sectors. The concept of Health Promotion which re-states the importance of policy and environmental action as well as individual behaviour change has been influential in moving from a victim blaming to a more conventional public health approach.

The revival of public health in towns and cities and the origins of the Healthy Cities Project

In the winter of 1985/86, the European office of the World Health Organization developed the proposal for a limited health promotion project, involving perhaps four to six cities and which would be known as the 'Healthy Cities Project'. The project was launched at an inaugural conference held in Lisbon in March 1986 and within a remarkably short time the notion of a project had become all but irrelevant. Towns and cities from around the world latched on to the idea of translating the WHO Health for All strategy (1981) and the thirty-eight European Targets for Health for All by the year 2000 (1985b) into local programmes. The underlying intention was to bring together a partnership of the public, private and voluntary sectors to focus on urban health and to tackle health-related problems in a broad way.

Many pre-existing strands of activity have come together to create this interest and in a sense the WHO initiative was pushing at an open door. Following the publication of the WHO Alma Ata declaration promoting the importance of Primary Health Care in 1978, initial progress in creating a new momentum for public health at the national level was slow despite the adoption of the Health for All Strategy by many countries. However, interest began to be expressed in the Health for All Strategy in an increasing number of health and local authorities. In Britain, the Mersey Regional Health Authority adopted a Health for All framework in 1984 and it was soon followed by Bloomsbury District Health Authority and many others. A British network of local authorities with health committees was established which became increasingly interested in the philosophy and framework offered by Health for All. Sheffield, Oxford and Nottingham were particularly quick to see the potential and to carry out special epidemiological studies of health in their areas, produce Health for All reports or initiate interventions aimed at promoting health, parallel initiatives were taking place as far apart as Toronto and Lisbon. In the voluntary sector a variety of self-help and community development projects which often had their origins in the social movements of the 1960s continued to develop and came to be seen as of increasing relevance and in particular the ideas of some of the ecological and green groups were being taken increasingly seriously.

A number of national governments, notably in Scandinavia, introduced legislation intended to reinforce the shift towards primary health care and commissioned reports focusing on Health for All. However, generally speaking there was frustration at the relative unwillingness of the medical sector to move towards a more social and less medical view of health.

Against this background a conference was held in Toronto in 1984 entitled 'Beyond Health Care', to review progress in public health in the ten years since the Lalonde Report had been published. One of the objectives of the conference was to shift the focus from victim blaming to healthy public policies. Somewhere in the ferment of ideas that year in Toronto, Len Duhl's notion of the Healthy City received an airing and it was readily picked up and taken back to WHO at Copenhagen by Dr Ilona Kickbusch, who saw in it an opportunity of translating the Health for All strategy into a tangible programme of action in which a few European cities would share their experiences with each other. A multidisciplinary steering group was convened and I was asked to co-ordinate the project from Liverpool University on behalf of WHO, drawing on the local experience and expertise developed as a result of implementing a Health for All Strategy in the Mersey Health Region together with the Regional Health Promotion Officer, Howard Seymour. Those experiences have been described elsewhere (Ashton and Seymour 1988).

Healthy Cities

The rationale for focusing on public health in towns and cities is strong. By the year 2000, 75 per cent of Europeans and the majority of the world's population will live in cities or large towns. Some Third World cities are expected to reach extremely large sizes by the end of the twentieth century: Mexico City, 31 million; São Paulo, 26 million; Rio de Janeiro, Bombay, Calcutta and Jakarta each exceeding 16 million; Seoul, Cairo and Manilla exceeding 12 million. The problems that were described in British cities 150 years ago are all to be found in these cities today, albeit on a much bigger scale and with much greater consequences. However, some things are different; technologies are available, such as immunization, which may enable some short-circuiting of the trajectory of intervention which was followed in Europe. Many of these cities have elaborate public sector organizations which may often be part of the problem in compartmentalizing their response to particular public health issues.

Increasingly, people are making the connection between the urban condition and the eco-crisis confronting the planet. According to the Chairperson of the World Commission on the Environment, Mrs Gro Harlem Bruntland (1987):

> There are also environmental trends that threaten to radically alter the planet, that threaten the lives of many species upon it, including the human species. Each year another 6 million hectares of productive dryland turns into worthless desert. Over three decades, this would amount to an area roughly as large as Saudi Arabia. More than 11 million hectares of forests are destroyed yearly, and this, over three decades, would equal an area about the size of India. Much of the forest is converted to low-grade farmland unable to support the farmers who settle it. In Europe, acid precipitation kills forests and lakes and damages the artistic and architectural heritage of nations; it may have acidified vast tracts of soil beyond reasonable hope of repair. The burning of fossil fuels puts into the atmosphere carbon dioxide, which is causing

gradual global warming. This 'greenhouse effect' may by early next century have increased average global temperatures enough to shift agricultural production areas, raise sea levels, to flood coastal cities, and disrupt national economies. Other industrial gases threaten to deplete the plant's protective ozone shield to such an extent that the number of human and animal cancers would rise sharply and the oceans' food chain would be disrupted. Industry and agriculture put toxic substances into the human food chain and into underground water tables beyond reach of cleansing.

There is an increasing realization throughout the world of the need to grapple with these self-induced crises which threaten global ecosystems. These crises are, in large part, the results of the lifestyle and expectations of city-dwellers and of the way in which they affect patterns of agriculture and world development. It is becoming apparent that some of the engineering solutions to the sanitary problems of cities cannot be adequately dealt with using Victorian approaches. In that sense the sanitary idea has been found wanting and incomplete. Moving sewage and solid waste away from its origin may work when a few comparatively small European cities are involved, but when a much greater proportion of a much bigger world population is implicated it is a recipe for ecological catastrophe as the carrying capacity of biological systems becomes overloaded. The refinement towards ecological from sanitary thinking has considerable implications for the way life is carried on in cities and for the policies which underpin it. However, the ecological idea of understanding how complex natural systems interact, and of working with them rather than attempting to subdue them, carries with it at least as powerful a motivational potential as the sanitary idea had in 1844. The challenge now is to move towards cities and towns which are based on sound ecological principles.

A recent workshop of environmental and public health professionals, meeting under the auspices of the World Health Organization in Liverpool, concluded that there is a need for a shared vision of the ecological city, and that such a vision should incorporate four principles (WHO 1988):

Minimum intrusion into the natural state   The principle of minimum intrusion requires that new development and restructuring should reflect the topographic, hydrographic, vegetal and climatic environment in which it occurs. A close reference to the natural site will benefit drainage, ventilation, insulation, the indoor climate, the micro-climate and open and green spaces.

Maximum variety   Maximum variety should be aimed for in the physical, social and economic structure of the city. Land uses and activities should be mixed where this does not create hazards, rather than separated and fragmented. A range of economic activities will make cities and communities less vulnerable to change and reduce social polarization and inequalities.

As closed a system as possible The principle of closed systems in urban and environmental health management would mean that waste is recycled within the urban area wherever possible, and that water, energy and resources are renewable. The management of green spaces would maintain nature and recreational opportunities within cities.

An optimum balance between population and resources Urban and population change must relate to the fragile natural systems and environments that support them. Balance is required at the city and neighbourhood levels to provide a high quality and supportive physical environment, as well as economic and cultural opportunities.

These principles and this approach have been underlined by the European Charter on Environment and Health (WHO 1989).

The WHO Project

The Healthy Cities Project began at a meeting of twenty-one European cities in Lisbon in 1986, when it was agreed to collaborate in developing sound approaches to city health. The focus of the WHO initiative is somewhat programmatic, and perhaps bureaucratic, working as it does around five major elements:

1 The formulation of concepts leading to the adoption of city plans for health which are action-based and which use Health for All, health promotion principles and the 38 European targets as a framework.
2 The development of models of good practice which represent a variety of different entry points to action depending on cities' own perceived priorities. These may range from major environmental action to programmes designed to support individual life-styles change, but illustrate the key principles of health promotion.
3 Monitoring and research into the effectiveness of models of good practice on health and cities.
4 Dissemination of ideas and experiences between collaborating cities and other interested cities.
5 Mutual support, collaboration and learning, and cultural exchange between the towns and cities of Europe.

In order to achieve these objectives, participating cities agreed to undertake seven specific tasks:

1 To establish a high-level, intersectoral group bringing together the executive decision makers from the main agencies and organizations within the city. The purpose of this group is to take a strategic overview of health in the city and unlock their organizations to work with each other at every level.
2 To establish an intersectoral officer or technical group as a shadow to the

executive group to work on collaborative analysis and planning for health in the city.

3 To carry out a community diagnosis for the city down to the small-area level, with an emphasis on inequalities in health and the integration of data from a variety of sources including the assessment of public perception of their communities and their personal health.

4 The establishment of sound working links between the city and the local institutions of education both at a school and higher education level. Links at the school level can be explored as partnerships for learning, at the higher education level as partnerships for research and teaching. These latter links should not be confined to medical training establishments but should include any department or institution with an interest in urban health-related phenomena. Part of this work involves the identification of appropriate urban health indicators and targets based on the Barcelona criteria:

- That they should stimulate change by the nature of their political visibility and punch through being sensitive to change in the short-term and being comparable between cities.
- That they should be simple to collect, use and understand, be either directly available now or available in a reasonable time at an acceptable cost.
- That they should be related to health promotion.

5 That all involved agencies should conduct a review of the health promotion potential of their activities and organizations, and develop the application of health impact statements as a way to make health promotion potential in different policy areas explicit. This includes the recognition that within a city there are many untapped resources for health, both human and material.

6 That cities will generate a great debate about health within their cities which involves the public in an open way and which works actively with the local media. This might include the generation of debate and dialogue using, for example, the interfaces which exist with the public, such as schools, community centres, museums, libraries and art galleries. A city's own public health history is itself often a powerful focus for debate and learning. Part of this work is the exploration of developing effective health advocacy at the city level.

7 The adoption of specific interventions aimed at improving health based on Health for All principles and the monitoring and evaluation of these interventions. The sharing of experience between cities and the development of multiple cultural links and exchanges underlies this work and is seen as promoting one fundamental goal of the World Health Organisation, i.e. the promotion of world peace and understanding without which all health is threatened.

The emphasis of these tasks is on the provision of enabling mechanisms for health promotion to be developed through healthy public policy and increased public accountability; it is also on breaking down vertical structures and barriers and obtaining much better horizontal integration for working together.

Nevertheless, buried within these can be found, to a greater or lesser extent, most of the activities of the local Health of Towns Association branches of 1844–5, bringing together key players in the cities, establishing a clear picture of health in different parts of the city, developing advocacy and coalition, building for change, intervention and legislation.

This volume represents an attempt to bring together some of the experiences of trying to develop a new urban public health. Some of the contributions have come from people who are involved with the WHO European project cities, others such as those from Australia, Canada and the United States are from sister initiatives which have derived their stimulus from the European initiative, yet others – in particular those from Valencia and from the Basque Country of Spain – are examples of pragmatic opportunism, linking the WHO idea to existing work.

The contributions from Marilyn Rice and from Trudy Harpham draw on extensive experience in the rapidly developing cities of the Third World. They bring a perspective which is seen to be of increasing importance as the immensity of the impact of urbanization on public health is being realized. It is hoped that the contributions taken as a whole are seen to provide a mosaic of ideas that might stimulate and support the work that is going on around the world.

Conclusion

The move from sanitary to ecological thinking has considerable implications for the ways in which we think about, plan and live in our towns and cities. However, the ecological idea of understanding how complex natural systems work, and of working with – rather than against – them is a challenge which Chadwick and his colleagues of the 1840s would surely have relished. In fact, Chadwick, who was in many ways ahead of his time, was already thinking along these lines himself. According to the introduction to the Edinburgh University edition of the Chadwick Report (published in 1965):

> mention ought to be made of one of the more curious bees in Chadwick's bonnet; his enthusiasm for the use of untreated sewage as a field manure. . . . he firmly believed that the sale of urban sewage to farmers in the neighbourhood of towns would wholly pay for the cost of sewerage, although it is only fair to add that Chadwick planned for the removal of sewage from the towns not in solid form, but by suspension in water. . . . To Chadwick, the emptying of sewers into rivers anywhere seemed like pouring away liquid gold.

The challenge to us is to pick up where Chadwick's thinking left off 100 years ago. Nor should we be fazed by those who regard ecology as a bee in a bonnet. The time is short, but there are many allies, and it is imperative that broad-based professional, public and political coalitions be built to tackle the problems which confront us.

It remains to be seen whether a global movement in the 1990s can be as effective as a national one in the 1840s.

Acknowledgements

I wish to acknowledge the contribution of Janet Ubido in carrying out research into the history of the Health of Towns Association and to Professor J. N. Morris who first put me on the right track (as usual).

Some parts of this chapter have previously been presented as the Chadwick Memorial Lecture at the 97th Annual Conference of the Institution of Environmental Health Officers of England.

References and further reading

Ashton, J. (1986) *Healthy Cities – Action Strategies for Health Promotion*. First and second WHO project brochures published by Liverpool University Department of Public Health.

Ashton, J. (1988) *Healthy Cities – Concepts and Visions*. A resource for the WHO Healthy Cities Project. Liverpool: Department of Public Health, University of Liverpool.

Ashton, J., Grey, P. and Barnard, K. (1986) 'Healthy Cities – WHO's New Public Health Initiative', *Health Promotion* 1(3):319–24.

Ashton, J. and Seymour, H. (1988) *The New Public Health*, Milton Keynes: Open University Press.

Ashton, J. (ed.) (1988) Proceedings of the first United Kingdom Healthy Cities Conference, Liverpool, 28–30 March. Published by Liverpool University Department of Public Health.

Ashton, J. (1991) 'Sanitarian becomes Ecologist: The New Environmental Health', *British Medical Journal* editorial 302: 189–90.

Ashton, J. and Ubido, J. (1991) 'The Healthy City and the Ecological Idea'. Paper presented at the Society for the Social History of Medicine. *Social History of Medicine* 4(1): 173–81.

Beyond Health Care (1985) Proceedings of a working conference on Healthy Public Policy, *Canadian Journal of Public Health* 76 (suppl.) 1–104.

Bruntland, G.H. (1987) *Our Common Future: The Report of the World Commission on Environment and Development*, Oxford: Oxford University Press.

Chadwick, E. (1965) [1842] *Report on the Sanitary Condition of the Labouring Population of Great Britain*, Introduction by M.W. Flinn, Edinburgh: Edinburgh University Press.

Chave, S. (1987) 'Recalling the Medical Officer of Health'. Edited by M. Warren and H. Francis, London: King Edward's Hospital Fund.

Duhl, L. (1986) 'The Healthy City: Its Function and its Future', *Health Promotion* 1: 55–60.

Finer, S.E. (1952) *The Life and Times of Sir Edwin Chadwick*, London: Methuen.

Hancock, T. (1986) 'Lalonde and Beyond: Looking Back at "A New Perspective on the Health of Canadians"', *Health Promotion* 1(1): 93–100.

Harpham, T., Lusty, T. and Vaughan, P. (1988) *In the Shadow of the City – Community Health and the Urban Poor*, Oxford: Oxford University Press.

Health of Towns Commission (1845) *Remedial Measures, Local Reports,* second report, volume 1, London: William Clowes and Sons.

Lalonde, M. (1974) *A New Perspective on the Health of Canadians,* Ottawa: Government of Canada.

Lewis, R.A. (1952) *Edwin Chadwick and the Public Health Movement 1832–1854,* London: Longmans Green and Co.

Liverpool Mercury (1845) Meeting of Inhabitants of Liverpool. Health of Towns Association, 25 April.

Lovelock, J. (1989) *The Ages of Gaia – A Biography of Our Living Earth,* Oxford: Oxford University Press.

McKeown, T. (1976) *The Role of Medicine – Dream, Mirage or Nemesis,* London: Nuffield Provincial Hospitals Trust.

Milio, N. (1986) *Promoting Health through Public Policy,* Ottawa: Canadian Public Health Association.

Tabibzadeh, I., Rossi-Espagnet, A. and Maxwell, R. (1989) *Spotlight on the Cities – Improving Urban Health in Developing Countries,* Geneva: WHO.

White, B.D. (1951) *History of the Corporation of Liverpool,* Liverpool: Liverpool University Press.

WHO (World Health Organisation) (1978) *Alma Ata. Primary Health Care,* Geneva: WHO.

WHO (1981) *Global Strategy for Health for All by the Year 2000,* Geneva: WHO.

WHO (1985a) *Health Promotion – A Discussion Document on the Concepts and Principles,* Copenhagen: WHO.

WHO (1985b) *Targets in Support of the European Strategy for Health for All,* Geneva: WHO.

WHO, Health and Welfare Canada, Canadian Public Health Association (1986) *Ottawa Charter for Health Promotion,* Copenhagen: WHO.

WHO (1988) 'Ecological Models for Healthy Cities Planning'. Report on WHO workshop, Liverpool, 25–27 March, Rapporteur P. Flynn, Copenhagen: WHO.

WHO (1989) *European Charter on Environment and Health,* Copenhagen: WHO.

Wohl, A.S. (1984) *Endangered Lives. Public Health in Victorian Britain,* London: Methuen.

I

Utopias and realities

2

Healthy Cities: myth or reality?

Len Duhl

The idea of Healthy Cities is basically a change in our way of thinking. Though the way is old, it has returned.

Simply put, it is an attempt to look at the whole of health and cities in relationship to its parts. Since the 1800s, when the focus was on particular causalities, we ignored the whole, what we could call CONTEXT as interfering with attaining the goal. This has been true for all fields, health not any different from others. From the earliest times traditional medical practice had a more holistic view than Western allopathic medicine. It is only recently that the complexity of health and medical issues has forced a systemic and ecological view (Duhl 1963; Ashton and Seymour 1988; DeLeuw 1989).

Many homogenous communities have, due to a strong religious value system, created holistic communities. Muslims, Jews, Buddhists and others have cosmologies which deal with all artefacts of life (Duhl 1988).

We see individual, family, organizational, urban, national and international health issues as complex interrelated systems that are ever changing. Though others focus on the new approach on other levels, we have chosen the city as the optimal one for intervention.

A city is hard to define. In the past, it had discrete boundaries and was a geographic entity, with a clear outline, demography and culture. Often, we noted a character of cities that made them unique: this remains. Now we see neighbourhoods, communities, cities, metropolis, and megalopolis as a phenomenon of urbanization. Urbanization is only in part an increase in density within a given geographic area. It includes a changing pattern of relationships and communication. Urbanization is expressed through culture, government, politics, the social and physical infrastructure and much more. It is also the overt replacement of the natural by a human-made environment.

One characteristic of this process, world-wide, is its diversity and its rapid growth. Thus, to intervene in health and urban processes with a systemic Healthy Cities approach, is to deal with a variety of people, institutions, values, cultures and more. The governance of this diversity is the most central issue in the programme. In innumerable cities the in-migration patterns bring diversity. San Francisco has twenty-six or more Asian cultures, sixteen Hispanic, and a variety of Black, European, and American Indian populations. Each bring with them beliefs, religions, values and health, nutrition, relationship and other practices. The dilemma is how to create a health programme that meets these multiple expectations. Do we try to persuade them to accept Western medicine? Can they use their own traditional practices? There are many unanswered questions.

One idea of Healthy Cities is that all separate programmes, groups and interests, *sit around a common table* to create a new holistic approach to health and other issues. This concern in an environmentally diverse context makes every situation unique, different and perhaps not recognizable to others. In many cities I learn through my visits of different people working in the same area. They have different points of view. One of my functions is to bring them together. Often, as happened in Shanghai, I introduced a planner and public health doctor to each other. Each had been working in the same area for many years without meeting. 'You know the Wu's and the Li's never talk!' I was thanked for the brokerage function.

The reality of Heathy Cities is that the process works some of the time. We would delude ourselves if we thought that every time we try to intervene it will be acceptable. Often the words are hailed, but the process is stymied. Sometimes the result is simply *old wine in new bottles*. One city I visited had a key official comment, 'We do not need a Healthy City programme. We have been a healthy city since the twelfth century!' Some cities say their programme on infant mortality are just what we have in mind. They add this to others that exist without the necessary interactive processes. Everything remains the same.

More often something starts, and it sputters along. The joy comes when the programme takes off and new patterns of solution emerge. In many communities, only the converted hear the message. Others are both oblivious and unaffected. In the gathering of people together it is hard to bring in the negative groups. Thus, only friends are part of the programme. It is a repeat of old discussions and nothing moves.

Why is this so? Change is a difficult process. In fact it is always going on, with events, often quite spontaneously, affecting the way things happen. Deliberate intervention has too often as its main outcome unintended consequences (Duhl 1986). A process starts towards a goal, and something else just happens to happen.

In the processes of gathering people together, the leader often has something in mind. Frequently, if the process is open, new ideas enter the dialogue. The group process comes out with ideas that had never been expressed. Often, when an official has said no, someone in the room finds that there is another solution. This process can go either way, and negative outcomes can arise. Linear change is a rare phenomenon. It occurs only when time is short, goals clear and scale small. Urban issues are instead complex, unclear, confused and ever changing. Change is full of ambiguous goals on multiple time lines. In fact, control of the intervention process is close to impossible. Who would have guessed that the changes in Eastern Europe would have occurred as they did? Here is an example where the future is full of ambiguities. People tend to extrapolate the present into the future and are surprised when something else happens. When a major change occurs, as in Eastern Europe, the future will be as much of a surprise as the early events. Be ready for new innovations.

Health in the last hundred years was based upon a *control* model. How to *control* illness? How to change and control behaviour? We have reached a moment in time where full control is impossible on every level. Families, institutions, governments and the world seem to many so out of control as to be disastrous. The words 'disease *control*' symbolize Public Health's past. If the top official plans, it is often an attempted process of getting people to agree with the formulation. When the leader asks others to participate the surprise leads to situations that threaten the position and authority of even the best of them.

We are in the process of creating a non-control model of change. Healthy Cities is both a response to and a cause of new control means of dealing with health. If all urban areas are diverse, and contain within them diverse groups, cultures, values and goals, a new means must emerge for responding to it. The values we have built into Health Promotion, Healthy Public Policy and Healthy Cities are such a response. For example, we respect diversity; we encourage participation and calls for equity, which asks that they sit together at a common table, explore the varied visions and create loosely coupled systems to respond.

The reality of many of our attempts to deal with health in cities is that they are full of process problems. How to involve people? What are new means for communicating? Are there possibilities of a common language for all the diverse groups? People have differing levels of experience. How can they teach each other? There was a time I found myself angry when people did not see the issue the way I did. I tried to convince, change, cajole and modify others. It doesn't work, unless there are means to *control*. One, of course, is power.

Many cities can hardly find one leader. They are collections of people. Money can aid control. However, we are in a time of a clear money deficiency. We have to find new sources, redirect what we have, and often live sparingly. *Control* is replaced by collaboration, and temporary coalitions. We have to talk, talk, talk and communicate. I have been asked about money in many of the cities. More and more communities report a shortage. However, as the problem is reframed, the opportunity to redirect available money appears. Most cities have found the resources in people, volunteer workers and in alternative money sources from groups never before involved in health issues.

'I cannot understand where you are!' 'Only I have the right perception of reality!' There are countless versions of resistance. However, most established bureaucracy is entrenched in the rewards it gets from the status quo. The hardest group to enervate is the middle civil service. Often the community and the top leadership clearly understand. It is the people doing their job repetitively and who feel good with what they have, who resist. No one gives up power spontaneously. Often it has to be wrested away.

What is significant is that resistance is important. It must exist. We must respect it. Only dialogue can help. In fact it might help each of us change our perceptions. The process of leadership (Gardner 1989; Bennis 1989) is the ability to aid in the process of reframing the problem. Though, *I* obviously know the correct new perception, *I* do not want to listen. To listen and hear means to move slowly into a win-win situation, rather than win-lose. In win-win there is a mediation of ideas, with concessions, change, synthesis and integration. More than anything it requires a new language.

The idea of teaching the community mediation techniques is important. In some cities where this has been done with adults and schoolchildren, there have been decreases in medical visits, contacts with the law, violence and crime. Conflict resolution may be more important than advocacy as a change tool. With fragmented communities that are diverse and cannot agree, they are like marriages and families in disarray. In dissolution the main topic is money. That has become the common language world-wide. Economics drives change, rather than change using the skill or economics and the nutrition of money to create activities. With a mediation model new language develops that all can understand. Rather than separate *games* being played, a *game of games* emerges. Syntheses can then occur.

Leaders of small programmes, what I like to call '*mamma-papa* stores', are quite competent to run programmes with small-scale dimensions. As the scale and complexity increase the infinite connections to the larger contextual environment, it requires new skills. These are political, though they connect to more than the governmental arena. It requires knowing a vast set of skills. They range from conceptualizing to planning, policy, administration, budget and financial management, consultation, and much more. This can be done by teams, since it is hard for one person to do it all. I have likened the difference between a *mamma-papa* store and a *supermarket* as a difference that is more than size. The latter requires understanding a large number of entrepreneurial and managerial techniques. A collection of many small stores doesn't make a supermarket. Learning of a new kind must occur. In many of the experimental and pilot programmes in Healthy Cities, the move from the small scale to the large policy arena has not taken place.

The reality that exists in most Healthy City programmes is that we have few social entrepreneurs (Duhl 1990) who have the skills to work in the larger arena. In many places, if the skills exist, coming from the business community, they do not have the values central to our work. Recruitment of potential social entrepreneurs requires a follow up of training, and continued support by colleagues (often in other Healthy City programmes).

I have run into a large number of people who came from other jobs and disciplines, who have had the values Healthy Cities profess but were unused. They, when given the opportunity, can transfer the metaphor from one field to another. For example, an advertising executive used his skills to market programs of nutrition and well baby care. He produced and wrote soap operas for local radio with both a story line and health messages.

(Manoff 1985)

The dilemma of training is that most occurs on the job. All too often the people involved are mostly the professionals. They have single track views, and little experience with teams, or multidisciplinary settings. I have often found that the housewife, trained perhaps unfairly to do a multiplicity of simultaneous tasks is better able to understand and work in complex urban settings than the skilled professional. The difference between the non-professional housewife and the so-called expert is the ability to respond to the immediate need, with a long-range context. The mother wants to deal both with a child's pain and with the rest of its life.

Continuing education, by consumer and fieldworker, is as important as that which comes from professional authorities. There is a difference between school education where an expert professes, and a community get together to learn. In the latter ideas come from everyone. All are experts, of different kinds. I am always surprised both with the broad vision and the expertise available in a community group. Blending with experts on a joint team produces extraordinary information and learning.

The temptation in many programmes has been to avoid the Healthy Public Policy issues. They are more difficult since they require skills of political ability that few health personnel have learned. Not only are systemic orientations important but also the ability to deal with unknown areas of power (Milio 1981).

Work in the larger arena, dealing with the social infrastructure, and political connections to all sectors can lead to burn out. Many people get very tired of the multiple meetings. It is difficult repeatedly to begin over again as new people join the endeavour. The sheer volume of activity and information required to keep up to date takes much time. Psychological and emotional support is important. Time off for busy workers is essential. Even the highest paid professionals need time to relax. The idea of the sabbath, or sabbaticals, permits bringing in ideas from new places. It should not be limited to professors.

We require information systems. Recently, Centerlink, a California information systems company, has developed a complex system. They can draw from a wide variety of databases in different fields. All users can, based on their needs, obtain instant full or partial text recall of a collection of information that is integrated and synthesized.

Fragmented information systems, as fragmented as the fields, are of little help. Working with them results in overload and anxiety. The changing patterns of libraries make them important partners. More than anything, informing the larger community is essential. I have been meeting the press around the world and find that they want quick crisis information. However, when offered the opportunity to get *the news behind the news*, after initial resistance, their hunger for synthesized information is almost insatiable. Regular briefings of reporters, editors and publishers is essential. For the past years I have participated in sessions with groups of the media. Bringing a few experts, consumers and people from other communities together, new learning takes place. Once convinced that the idea of Healthy Cities is an important one, the media can pass on the idea better than professionals. Many reporters sit on unpublished information about cities which are valuable to us. Again, the process involves equitable partnership.

Without evaluation and feedback no programme can really continue (Duhl and Hancock 1988). There are many ways to assess progress. Hard data are important. So are stories, anecdotes, and anthropological and journalistic reports on who is doing what to whom.

I have outlined a set of realities of work in Healthy Cities areas. Each reader can fill in the details with a myriad of examples. We need to have information on how all programmes are dealing with these issues. There are many myths in this work. For many, 'It can't work!' For others, 'This is the greatest, best and most effective programme!' Still others pour our unsubstantiated positive and negative anecdotes. What is needed is to turn the whole Healthy City programme into a university in dispersion, where the walls come down, and the community educates itself. It has been said that Healthy Cities is a movement. I have suggested that it is the passing on of a health infection, a virus if you will, which allows cities to take from it what they can, and create their unique programme (Duhl and Webb n.d.). Like the DNA of a virus, the Healthy City ideas combine with the local DNA (its way of being) and produces new ways of running this health programme. We have shifted from the old notion of power as control to influence and collaboration. In some ways there is no such thing as a Healthy City. Each city is struggling in a variety of ways to reach a unique vision that they have.

The myth is that we can know what each city will achieve. It also is a myth that all will succeed. In fact, cities may have to find their own path, with their own non-Healthy Cities label. If they see their city as theirs, and not just a place they happen to be in, they will achieve their ends.

For those of us who believe that health, holism, holy, healing and whole are similar, Healthy Cities offers us a chance to bring all our own separate parts together as we help our own cities.

References

Ashton, J. and Seymour, H. (1988) *The New Public Health*, Milton Keynes: Open University Press.
Bennis, W. (1989) *On Becoming a Leader*, New York: Addison Wesley.

DeLeuw, E. (1989) *The Same Revolution – Health Promotion*, Copenhagen: WHO.

Duhl, L. (1963) *The Urban Condition*, New York: Basic Books.

Duhl, L. (1986) *Health Planning and Social Change*, New York: Human Sciences Press.

Duhl, L. (1988) 'The Mind of the City – The Context for Urban Life', *Environments* 19(13): 1–13.

Duhl, L. (1990) *The Social Entrepreneurship of Change*, New York: Pace University Press.

Duhl, L. and Hancock, T. (1988) 'Community Self-Evaluation – A Guide to Assessing Healthy Cities', *Healthy Cities Papers*, Copenhagen: FADL.

Duhl, L. and Webb, M. (n.d.) 'Some Lessons on Project Development for "Healthy Cities" – A Collaboration of "Virus and Cell"', unpublished paper.

Gardner, J. (1989) *On Leadership*, Gencoe, Ill: Free Press.

Manoff, R. (1985) *Social Marketing*, New York: Praeger.

Milio, N. (1981) *Promoting Health through Public Policy*, Philadelphia: F.A. Davis.

3

The Healthy City: Utopias and realities

Trevor Hancock

The Healthy City concept challenges cities with two seemingly simple questions: what is a healthy city and how do we get one? It is the attempt to answer the first question that takes us into the realm of Utopias; it is the response to the second that brings us face to face with reality.

The notion of utopian thinking has got what the Americans would call 'a bum rap'! Somehow, the term has come to mean hopelessly idealistic, airy-fairy, 'pie in the sky' thinking that ignores the 'real' world. That is because we have misconstrued the role of utopian thinking. Good utopian thinking provides us with a beacon to light our way forward and a goal to strive to achieve; it also tells us what we would like the world to be like, as opposed to what we think it will be like.

In the serious business of futurism and strategic planning, key activities of all major institutions in society today, including government and business, utopian thinking is more often referred to in terms of 'visions', 'preferable futures', 'scenarios' and 'goals'. But what they are talking about, beneath all the technical jargon, is nothing more nor less than utopian thinking, allied to a clear and pragmatic process of planning and operating strategically, of figuring out how to get from here to there.

Envisioning the future

John Naisbitt, an American futurist and author of *Megatrends* (1984), has noted:

> Strategic planning is worthless unless there is first a strategic vision...
> which guides every step of the process.
>
> (Naisbitt 1984)

The first vital step in futures/strategic planning, then, is to develop a vision of what the preferable future should be like, then develop that into an easily understood and plausible scenario and use that as a goal.

A vision is just that, a visual image in our mind's eye of what the situation would look like if everything we could wish for came to pass; in this case, if our city or community could be as healthy as possible. This process of developing a vision can be done fairly easily in small or even large groups, using a technique known as 'guided imagery' in which people are led, or guided, through a process of seeing in their mind's eyes, or envisioning, the way things should be.

A few years ago, such an idea might well have been looked upon as a rather weird thing to do, definitely a bit 'new age' and suspect, but today it is a well-accepted technique used by management consultants and planners in all sorts of settings. One of the best known ways of using this process has been in the sports area, where athletes are taught to 'see' themselves playing the perfect stroke, or making the perfect pass, or clearing the high jump bar, before they go out and do it. The same idea is also used with cancer patients, who are taught to see their bodies successfully fighting off and defeating their cancer.

In the case of the Healthy City Projects, groups of people are taken through the process of envisioning their city as ideally healthy and then those individual visions are combined in various ways to arrive at a commonly shared vision which is then written down as a story or 'scenario' describing the vision in easily understood, everyday terms. (See T. Hancock in *Healthy Cities – Concepts and Visions* (1988), published by the Department of Public Health at Liverpool University, for details of the envisioning process and an example of a scenario.)

We also need to keep in mind that within any city or town, there will be varying views of what constitutes a healthy city. Thus it is important in putting together 'Vision Workshops' to make them as multisectoral as possible, and if possible also to ensure they have a good mix of the different social and ethnic groups in the city. Alternatively, separate workshops should be organized for these different groups. In the end, the scenario is based on the input from all those groups, ending up with a richer and more representative vision, though still one that emphasizes the commonality of a shared vision.

The uniqueness of a vision

It is important to recognize that each community or city should go through this exercise itself and not just adopt some other city's vision. This is because every city or community will have its own understanding of health and its own unique circumstances. For example, when I conducted a vision workshop with a group in the Australian capital city of Canberra, two of the elements of a Healthy City that emerged were, in my experience, unique.

The first was actually a missing element: there was very little emphasis on the quality of the physical environment in their vision, unlike anywhere else I have known. The second was the strong emphasis on local democracy as a central element of their vision. The reason for these unique elements is in the very nature of Canberra. As the Commonwealth (federal) capital, it was built from scratch in the early part of this century, and was a fairly small place until quite recently. There was no primary industry (hence, not a lot of pollution), generally good and modern housing and the whole city is well planned and laid out in a very attractive natural setting. Clearly, they have for the most part achieved a fairly healthy physical environment.

Not so for their social environment. The business of the city is government, it is a fairly new city, it has a mobile population and as a result there is a lack of strong social networks. Even worse, it has been from the start a federal capital on federal land, administered by the Minister and the bureaucracy responsible for the Territories. There was until very recently no directly elected City Council or Mayor and thus it is not surprising that there would be a sense that people lacked control over the conditions and events of city life that shaped their health and well-being.

While not every city will have such a unique vision of a Healthy City, this example does serve to remind us that every city and every community is unique.

A preferable future

The key point about the vision that is generated is that it is an example of the preferable future. It is equally possible, of course, to have people imagine a very unhealthy future, or as is more often the case, to have them envision the probable future.

The distinction between probable and preferable futures is an important one, because often what we think is most likely to happen – nuclear war or the 'greenhouse effect' for example – is not at all what we would like to have happen, so we prefer to ignore unpleasant possibilities and focus on the familiar and the optimistic. Thus much of our planning and most of our daily lives are built on the assumption that the probable future will be very much like today, only more so. We tend to imagine the future, very often, as 'more of the same' or 'business as usual', or what is sometimes called 'the official future'.

This is perhaps inevitable; we would find it hard to plan and lead our lives if we knew only that tomorrow would be completely different from today, but didn't know in what way it would be different. We have to assume that it will be the same, or pretty nearly so. But the problem with such an approach is that it doesn't allow for and certainly doesn't encourage much change. On the contrary, the image of the probable future we carry in our individual and collective minds tends to encourage us to work to keep things the way they are. And when we see things getting worse, it tends to paralyse us, if we can't imagine a better alternative. Creating a vision of a preferable future, then, becomes very important when things are not going well. It holds out the hope that things could perhaps be better, and encourages us to find ways of changing things so that we can create such a future, or at least a future closer to the one we prefer than the one we fear is probable.

Muddling towards Utopia

It is in the attempt to figure out how to get from 'here' to 'there' that futurism becomes strategic planning. It also helps us understand the importance of what the British futurist James Robertson said: 'thinking about the future is useful and interesting only if it affects what we do and how we live today' (1988).

The shared vision of a Healthy City – expressed as a scenario, or pictures or a video or any other way that is useful – becomes the goal for which the city and its people strive. In this sense, a goal is a timeless statement of aspiration, something we are always striving to achieve but can never quite reach. But while our ultimate goal will not change, how we work to attain that goal will likely change over time. That is because as time passes, our environment changes, as do our social values, our scientific and technological possibilities and, perhaps most important, our political and community realities.

For this reason, we should be very suspicious of master plans that will, supposedly, bring us to our goal in ten or twenty years. In an era of unprecedented change, it is very difficult, if not impossible, to be able to forecast what the world will be like. In the mid-1980s who would have foreseen the dramatic changes in Eastern Europe in 1989. Once such changes – what futurists call a discontinuity – have occurred, we are in a different reality. The master plans devised in 1988 were out of date by 1990!

So instead of trying to develop a master plan for attaining a Healthy City that will in all probability join all the other master plans on the bookshelf, we need a process of 'goal (or vision) directed muddling through'. In other words, once we are clear where we are going, then we should be flexible and innovative, taking advantage of every opportunity to move forwards, but being prepared to move sideways – or even to take a step backwards if our way is blocked – if that's what it takes to get where we are trying to go.

Muddling through has, like Utopia, developed a bad name. But just as utopian thinking is of no value if you don't have a clear idea of how you are going to get there, so muddling through is of no value as a strategy if you don't know where you are trying to go. As the Cheshire Cat said to Alice in *Alice's Adventures in Wonderland*: 'if you don't know where you want to go, it really doesn't matter which path you take' (Carroll 1954). And most of the time, muddling through is for the sake of muddling through, with no clear sense of direction. Under such circumstances, it is not likely you will get very far and nobody will be impressed by your efforts.

In order to muddle through effectively or to figure out strategy to get us from where we are now to where we want to be, we need to do some strategic planning. This will help us identify opportunities for inspired muddling through, as well as threats to be avoided. This is done through a process called 'environmental scanning'.

Environmental scanning

The environment to be scanned has two components: the external environment of the group or organization and its internal environment. The external environment should be scanned in a number of major categories:

1 social issues
2 environment/ecology
3 economics
4 politics
5 technology.

'Scanning' basically involves looking at these categories, trying to get a handle on what are the major trends and issues and figuring out what threats they pose or what opportunities they present as you attempt to move towards your preferable future.

The scan should involve all seemingly relevant issues at the local, regional, national, international and global levels. Obviously, such an undertaking could be an enormous task, keeping lots of people fully occupied for months. For large corporations, this may indeed be the case. On the other hand, for a Healthy City Project, it may mean having a city staff person work on it part-time for a few months, in conjunction with a multisectoral steering group, or it may mean no more than asking some local experts to meet with the Healthy City steering group for a day and identify some key issues in their own area of expertise. For a small community group it could be done equally well by sitting around one evening and kicking some ideas around, within a simple framework, such as that shown in Table 3.1.

Table 3.1   Simple framework for environmental scanning

	Key issues/trends	*Opportunity threat*
Social issues		
Environment/ecology		
Economics		
Politics		
Technology		

Obviously, the more resources you have, the more complex and sophisticated will be the product. However, that can also be a disadvantage because the amount of detail may become overwhelming and you will miss the wood for the trees. Or, to use a better analogy, you want only a cheap and simple radar system that will stop you flying into the tops of the mountains, not one that will give you a detailed picture of the terrain of the foothills.

The internal analysis is equally important but is one that, perhaps understandably, we are often reluctant to perform for it is seldom very flattering. We need to know the strengths and weaknesses of our own organization in terms of:

1 People
   - number
   - quality
   - skills
   - adaptability
2 Funds/resources
   - adequacy
   - appropriate allocation
3 Organizational structure and culture
   - flexibility
   - quality of management
   - commitment to a goal.

Again, this can be either a simple or a complex process, and again, the simpler one may prove better.

A strategic plan

Once you know where you are going, what opportunities and threats you face and what human and other resources you can muster, you are ready to develop a strategic plan. Again, this can be either a fairly simple or a very complex process; simplicity is often best.

You need a clear and agreed upon *mission statement* which tells the world – and more importantly your own organization – what business you are in, for example, 'We play a leadership role in making our city as healthy as possible.'[1]

Next, you want a set of *strategic priorities* that suggest how you will do this; not too many, four to six will do, for example:
We shall

1 reduce inequities in health opportunities
2 create physical environments that support health
3 create social environments that support health
4 strengthen the community's capacity, ability and opportunity to take action to protect and improve their health

5 help people develop the skills they need to be healthy
6 reorientate our health services towards health promotion, disease prevention and community-based care.

From this point, you can then proceed to outline what specific *actions* you will take, how, and with whom, to achieve your purpose. This ought to include specifying quantifiable, achievable, time-limited *objectives* such as:

> by 1995, we will have reduced the proportion of unfit housing from 10 per cent of our housing stock to 2 per cent.

This level of planning, of course, requires good knowledge of what the situation is and what is achievable, and can be a very time-consuming, but worthwhile, process.

Summary

If we are to make our cities more healthy, we need a clear vision of what our preferable future will be like, as a guide to our actions. Having then considered the opportunities and threats in our social, environmental, economic, political and technological environments and the strengths and weaknesses of our own organization, we can create a clear strategic plan that outlines the priority areas for action. Thus we can hope to move realistically towards our utopian future through a process of vision-directed muddling through.

Note

1 This mission statement and the four strategic priorities which follow it are based on those contained in *Healthy Toronto 2000* (published by the City of Toronto) and reflect the *Ottawa Charter for Health Promotion*, published by the the World Health Organisation (Copenhagen) in 1986.

References and further reading

Amara, R. (1981) 'The Futures Field', *The Futurist* 15(1): 25–9; 15(2): 63–71; 15(3): 42–6.
Carroll, L. (1954) *Alice's Adventures in Wonderland*, London: Macmillan (first published 1865).
Cassedy, J. (1962) 'Hygeia: A Mid-Victorian Dream of a City of Health', *Journal of the History of Medicine* 17(2): 217–28.
Cornish, E. (ed.) (1979) *The Study of the Future*, Washington, DC: World Future Society.
Hancock, T. (1985) 'An Introduction to Health Futurism', *Health Management Forum* 6(1): 17–25.
Hancock, T. (1988) 'Healthy Toronto 2000: A Vision of a Healthy City' in *Healthy Cities – Concepts and Visions*. A resource for the WHO Healthy Cities Project. Liverpool: Department of Public Health, University of Liverpool.

Naisbett, J. (1984) *Megatrends: Ten New Directions Transforming Our Lives*, London and Sydney: Future Macdonald.

Richardson, B.W. (1875) *Hygeia: A City of Health*, London.

Robertson, J. (1988) *The Future of Cities, Economic Choices and Possibilities*. Proceedings of the first United Kingdom Healthy Cities Conference, Liverpool. Edited by Dr J. Ashton and L. Knight, Liverpool: Department of Public Health, University of Liverpool.

4

Measuring health in cities

Peter Flynn

The measurement of 'health' in Britain has been dominated by two traditions of research. One focuses on the relationship between health and class (or social status). The other has examined the geographical relationship between health and measures of income, poverty or deprivation. The latter have been the basis for measuring the relative health of cities, and of different types of social areas within them.

Both types of research have shown a strong association between poor health and low income and social status. This is not surprising given the concentration of particular groups in types of cities, and in areas within them. These two traditions have been brought together in a number of studies, the best known of which was the report in 1980 of a government-appointed Research Working Group on *Inequalities in Health*, commonly known as the Black Report. The report received wide coverage because of its conclusion that poverty or material deprivation was highly correlated or associated with ill health. This relationship was reflected in variations in health characteristics between regions and health authorities, and suggested that health policies should reflect the influence of the wider variations of income, housing conditions, and other health determinants between groups and areas.

The national picture published in the Black Report (1980) and updated in 1987 has been confirmed in a number of local 'Black Reports', which describe the variations in health between small areas within cities. Studies have been carried out for a large number of cities including London, Sheffield, Manchester, Bristol and Liverpool. These studies use similar data because of the limited amount of information available to measure health inequalities for small areas of cities. In particular there is a heavy reliance on mortality data and particularly standardized mortality ratios.

The Standardized Mortality Ratio (SMR) is a measure used to allow comparisons of death-rates in different areas which takes account of the differences in age structure between them. Otherwise places with a high proportion of elderly people, such as the south coast retirement towns, would have consistently higher death-rates than other areas, but which did not reflect variations relating to differences in income and material conditions. The SMR is calculated by dividing the population into age groups and calculating for each of them the number of deaths which would occur if national age-specific death-rates were applied. The total number of expected deaths resulting from adding age group totals is then divided by the number of deaths actually recorded, and multiplied by 100.

If the resulting ratio is over 100, it shows that the area has an excess of deaths over nationally predicted rates. Conversely a figure of less than 100 shows that the area is experiencing less mortality than predicted from national rates. Standardized Mortality Ratios for those under 65 years of age are frequently used because they identify premature mortality.

This has the benefit of avoiding early 'excess' deaths being swamped in the overall ratio by the much greater number of deaths after 65. Additionally deaths at an early age are more easily ascribed to a specific cause whereas in old age there may be a range of illnesses, of which one has to be chosen as the cause of death.

Figure 4.1 shows the Standardized Mortality Ratios for Liverpool relative to national rates. It shows that for all causes of death for persons of all ages,

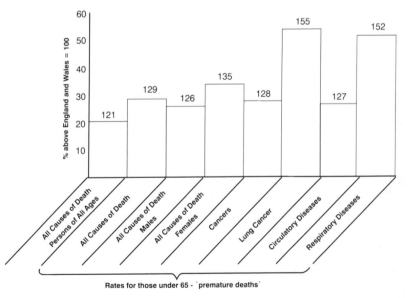

Figure 4.1 Standardized Mortality Ratios: Liverpool compared with the national SMRs.

there were 21 per cent more deaths than if national rates had applied. For premature deaths the figure was 29 per cent, and for specific causes of death, higher still. For lung cancer and respiratory diseases there were over 50 per cent more deaths than if national rates applied.

Figure 4.2 shows the range of SMRs within Liverpool's thirty-three electoral wards. It illustrates that the variation is wider than that between the Liverpool and national rates. It confirms the need for small area data to describe variations in health within cities to

1 describe the processes which produce group and area inequalities
2 establish priorities for action and to target resources
3 monitor the impact of changes over time
4 integrate data and provide the context for surveys and research
5 provide a framework for the evaluation of models of good practice
6 allow cities to exchange experiences on the basis of group and area effects.

Mortality is a frequently used measure of health because of its availability for small areas, and the fact that it is regularly published. Other measures which are used include infant mortality and low-birth-weight babies. Factors such as permanent sickness and disability provide good measures but are available only every ten years from national Censuses of Population.

In a number of areas studies have been carried out which allow a more systematic analysis of the relationship between health and poverty or deprivation. These have been based on a study (Townsend, Philimore and Beattie

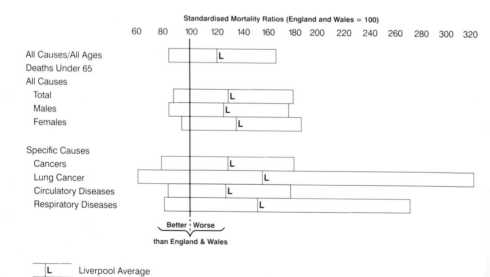

Figure 4.2 Standardized Mortality Ratios within Liverpool: the range of SMRs within the thirty-three wards.

1986) carried out for the Northern Health Region by the Health Authority and the University of Bristol. The studies use two indices, one to provide an overall health measure, and a second to describe deprivation.

The health index is made of three indicators: premature mortality, permanently sick or disabled residents, and low-birth-weight babies. The index is intended to provide a measure of health which reflects the health outcomes of present and past conditions. The deprivation measure is made up of four measures: unemployment, car ownership, non-owner-occupiers, and overcrowded households.

These measures were selected to reflect material deprivation through low income, a lack of 'wealth', and poor housing conditions. Figure 4.3 shows the relationship between the health and deprivation scores on these indices for each of the thirty-three electoral wards in Liverpool. It illustrates the strong association between health status and deprivation.

Even with analyses which cover one dimension of health status and processes, such as health and deprivation measures, there is considerable debate about the choice of appropriate indicators. There are a number of criteria which need to be adopted to ensure that indicators are relevant to studies of particular dimensions:

1 They should be direct measures of the problem. Unemployment, for example, or Standardized Mortality Ratios directly measure a dimension for which a policy response is required. The elderly or large families are indirect measures in that there are considerable variations within these groups in characteristics. Measures such as housing tenure are even less direct but have a value in interpreting the position of areas.
2 Where possible it should be clear what dimension of a problem or characteristic is being measured, i.e. low skill levels, low income, or low educational achievement.
3 The indicator should be consistent between areas. Sharing accommodation, for example, is a different experience for young professionals in parts of London compared with low-income families in other parts of the inner city.
4 The indicators should be consistent over time. The focus for housing problems has changed significantly in recent years. With the sale of council housing and policies to encourage owner-occupation amongst low income groups, tenure is no longer a good measure of relative housing status.
5 There should be a wide distribution of the characteristic and a large number of cases. One health measure used, infant mortality, is difficult to analyse for small areas because of the small number of cases, unless they are aggregated over a number of years.
6 The indicators should have a clear meaning and significance. It is vital for their use that the trends and distributions represented by indicators are understood, including by community groups, if they are to stimulate change.
7 The indicators should be easily available at a low cost, if they are to be used in a variety of areas to allow comparisons.

The use of the measures and techniques described above allows the mapping and analysis of health inequalities both between and within cities. There are issues in relation to the types of areas for which analyses are carried out, how far they reflect the variations between the health of groups within them, and the validity of the measures. In general, however, they are now widely used by cities in Britain and Europe to provide an initial analysis of health

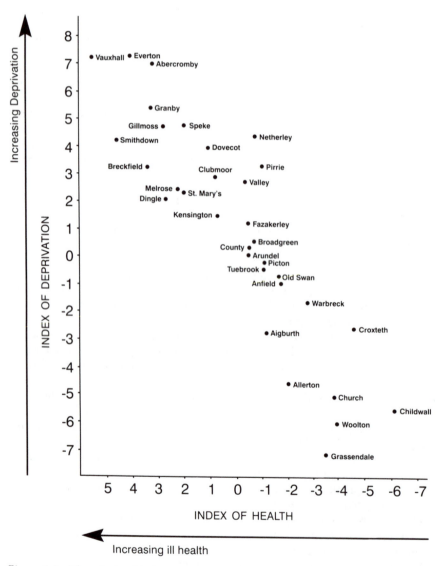

Figure 4.3   The relationship between deprivation and health scores on each index for the city's thirty-three wards.

inequalities, as a basis for setting targets and establishing priorities. Combined with information on the area's population and other characteristics they are often used to produce health 'profiles' of areas within cities.

A fundamental issue, particularly in relation to health promotion activities such as the Healthy Cities Project, is the lack of a conceptual framework for these studies. They raise the question of what is health, or a healthy city, and how can these concepts be measured?

The studies already described can be seen to measure not health but ill health or even death. There is an emphasis on negative measures which tend also to suggest explanations of health differences which relate to individuals, rather than wider groups or social processes. The problem is that while it is possible to develop concepts of health and social processes which are useful in policy terms, they are difficult to measure. Consequently the studies which are done use indicators which are easily measured but conceptually inadequate.

To illustrate the point in relation to individual health, it is worth looking at the possible progression from negative to positive measures. The most negative measure is mortality because it ignores the living altogether, although it is a health outcome which summarizes a wide range of health determinants. Premature deaths by specific causes are useful measures to provide a policy context. Morbidity or illness measures such as permanent sickness or disability are negative indicators, which in general identify physical, mental, or social disturbances. Such measures could be enhanced by the use of indicators of physical and functional characteristics such as height, weight, blood pressure, cholesterol level, physical fitness, hearing, and sight. In general such information is not available nationally to allow an analysis between and within cities. Methods have been developed, such as the Nottingham Health Profile, which measures subjective assessments of health on a range of dimensions covering pain, social isolation, physical mobility, energy, emotional reactions, and sleep.

The Profile identifies a minority of the population with what are essentially negative health experiences. It does, however, begin to approach the issue of health potential by allowing an analysis of change over time in perceived health status.

Definitions of health which begin to focus on positive concepts include 'an absence of illness, disease, and disability', and 'a state of complete, physical, mental, and social well-being'. These are essentially static measures and in the latter case are hard to imagine far less operationalize. More dynamic measures are required which relate to the concepts of health balance and potential. Balance suggests biological, psychological and social states which allow individuals to function effectively. Potential implies the opportunity to exploit one's health capacity, and to re-establish it when it is lost or threatened. People in quite different 'objective' health states, ranging from disability to an absence of any symptoms of illness, can be defined in terms of balance and potential which are useful in expressing positive concepts of current status and future change. One definition which has been put forward is that 'a person's health is equivalent to the state and set of conditions which fulfil or enable a person to work to fulfil his or her realistic chosen and biological potentials' (Seedhouse 1986).

How can these ideas be applied to the definition of 'Healthy Cities'? The World Health Organization's Healthy Cities Project involves a range of cities which have very different health, social, economic, and physical characteristics. On the negative measures and analyses of health described earlier in this chapter, cities such as Liverpool and Barcelona are clearly unhealthy cities in comparison with Stockholm and Rennes. They have higher levels of premature mortality and sickness which can be clearly associated with higher levels of poverty and deprivation. Within a project concerned with health promotion policies, however, it is important to identify the dynamics which will contribute to, or undermine, the overall objective of reducing inequalities in health.

Otherwise the fatalistic conclusion is that Healthy Cities are affluent cities and unhealthy ones are poor ones. In policy terms this provides no useful framework for exploiting the contribution which can be made by all the cities to achieving 'Health for All'. The concepts of balance and potential can be applied to cities as well as individuals. In this case we would be looking to the social, economic, physical and other conditions which provide the foundation for groups and individuals to be able to lead healthy and fulfilling lives.

Liverpool provides a classic example of the relationship between wider urban change, public policies, and the health of the city and its residents. It experienced very rapid growth in the nineteenth century as its population and economy grew dramatically.

The large number of in-migrants were housed in overcrowded and unsanitary housing. The combination of poverty, pollution, and poor living conditions led to high infant mortality rates and low life expectancy, primarily because of infectious diseases. The public policy response was based as much on fear of the spread of infectious disease as on altruism but helped give birth to the 'old public health' which recognized the wider causes of health as against narrow medical interventions. The provision of clean water, effective sewage, disposal systems, municipal housing, and later the clean air legislation, fundamentally improved the health of the residents. As important were the national social measures which increased people's incomes, and as a consequence improved their diet.

The responses were to a system which was out of balance because the social and physical infrastructure could not satisfy the needs of a growing and disadvantaged population. During the twentieth century Liverpool has experienced a similar lack of balance because of rapid population and economic decline. Since 1961 the city's population has fallen by over one-third and the number of jobs has almost halved. The migration from the city has been selectively of the younger and more skilled, leaving a concentration of the unemployed and low income groups. The health risks now are not infectious diseases, but those related to lifestyle. Smoking, poor diet, alcohol and drug abuse, and lack of exercise, are as systematically related to poverty and low income, as are smoking and ill health.

The public policy challenge is again to create a public health movement which recognizes the wider causes of health status, and the need for action at a variety of levels. At the European level the importance of acknowledging the concepts of balance and potential for cities has been demonstrated by studies of the relationship between population and employment change, and concentrations of groups which experience economic, social and health problems.

There are two groups of cities which experience high levels of deprivation and poor health. One group comprises cities and urban regions experiencing population decline.

They are predominantly the older industrial regions of Northern Europe, where the decline of industrial and port-related economies has led to high levels of unemployment and a skills base inappropriate to the economy of the 1990s. Four of the six urban regions with the highest levels of problems are British, and in Europe in general, ports are heavily represented.

The second group are predominantly Southern European cities undergoing a transition from an agrarian to an industrial economy. They are characterized by low incomes, high unemployment, and structural under-employment. As with Liverpool in the nineteenth century they experience stress in the provision of social and physical infrastructure because of their rapid urbanization. They face the same dangers of pollution and environmental degradation which will affect their ability to attract the new economic activities of the 1990s.

The creation of a single European market (1992) reinforces the trends which have seen a widening of the gap between the social and health status of cities, unless there are effective policy responses. The decline of the agricultural and manufacturing sectors, and the rise of the service sector, has seen a flow of people and jobs since the 1960s from larger Northern European cities to smaller ones and medium-sized towns. The process has more recently become apparent in Southern Europe.

The result has been a shift of economic activity and population to towns and cities in growing regions with low unemployment and high income levels. These are areas which are developed but have not suffered from dependence on declining industrial activities. They have high-quality environments, good communications, and are favoured locations for the profitable expanding service and high technology industrial sectors.

Their economies, population growth, and social and environmental infrastructure are 'in balance' and allow them to develop their potential as attractive places in which to live and work. Examples of these regions are the Alpine belt and Mediterranean France and they include 'successful' cities such as Grenoble, Nice and Montpellier.

By contrast the cities experiencing imbalanced change, either of growth or decline, are characterized by growing poverty, inequality and social polarization, financial crisis and deteriorating environments. There is evidence that older cities such as Glasgow can regenerate themselves by exploiting their cultural capital and attracting new service functions, including tourism. In these and more transitional cities such as London, however, the benefits of regeneration and adaptation have not extended to all groups and areas. In London, for example, the growth of poverty and the extreme of homelessness and ill health are the result of certain groups incurring the social costs of regeneration through their inability to afford basic requirements such as housing. Even the most prosperous cities have concentrations of the poor, but in theory at least have the overall resources to cure their own problems.

What factors therefore do we need to measure to identify progress towards achieving Healthy Cities' objectives in the very different contexts for different types of cities?

The first factor is the current health status of groups and areas. It has been shown earlier that measures are available, even though they focus on negative health, which do allow an analysis of health inequalities within areas. Attempting to bridge the gap between the concepts of balance and potential for healthy cities and individuals illustrates the importance of social processes in determining the health status of individuals and groups. The second factor, which needs to be measured is the range of health resources available to individuals and groups, which influences their behaviour and lifestyle and therefore their state of health. The basic resources cover elements such as employment and income, housing, and clean air and water. The resource also covers cultural and social values which influence the third factor to be measured, health behaviour.

Health behaviour can be positive through choosing a healthy diet, taking regular exercise, and using preventive health services. It can be negative through smoking, alcohol and drug abuse, and neglecting exercise, and preventive health treatment.

These social health resources and processes are heavily influenced by the wider social and economic conditions in cities, and by public policies. The fourth factor to be measured therefore is the overall balance, already referred to, between economic, demographic, social, and environmental conditions in cities and the way it is changing. This establishes the broad urban framework within which the fifth factor, public policy, operates.

The basic questions to be answered therefore are the following:

1 What are the overall conditions in the city?
2 What are the main features of public policy?
3 How do these two factors influence the health resources available to groups and their lifestyle?
4 What is the resulting state of health of individuals and groups and what are the appropriate policy interventions?

The Healthy Cities Project is an attempt to achieve a significant policy change in the way we address health problems. It moves from medical and individual explanations of health to preventive and social explanations. As such it needs to influence policy at a variety of levels from the international down to that of the local community.

The objectives of the European Commission's regional policy specifically refer to the 'balanced' development of regions to exploit their growth 'potential', and to reduce disparities. As part of this process objectives exist to ease the costs of adjustment especially for the poorer residents of larger cities, and to assist cities in changing their economic and social roles by improving their attractiveness as places to live and work. National policies are required which recognize the importance of achieving the urban regeneration and adjustment which benefits all groups and particularly those with low health status. National policies on economic development, housing, transport, and education all have group and area effects, and health dimensions and consequences.

In addition to making explicit the health dimension of a wide range of policies there are of course specific health promotion programmes. These include environmental health measures which reduce hazards and health threats, the development of good primary health care provision, and health promotion programmes which encourage changes in lifestyle. The experience of some health promotion programmes illustrates the need for effective evaluation of the impact of policies.

Campaigns can actually widen the gap between the health status of groups, where they are predominantly taken up by more affluent people with the income and resources and therefore choice to exploit them and achieve improvements in health and lifestyle.

Nevertheless there are examples of local projects and policies in every city which empower individuals and groups, and achieve improvements in health. A healthy city is one in which the conditions exist or are being created to allow people to exploit the potential which exists in every individual and location.

Measurement and evaluation are central tasks for those involved in the Healthy Cities movement. The programme has as central objective, the reduction of health inequalities, but is becoming established at a time when health and other inequalities between groups and between cities are growing. We need visions to achieve Healthy Cities. These visions, however, need to be available to all groups and we need to be sure that they are being or will be achieved.

Effective measurement and evaluation are very often the neglected activities within any project. This is even more the case where the task is as complex as the one which has been outlined. Measures do not exist which cover the range of factors identified as being necessary to evaluate progress towards achieving healthy city objectives. Very often they are inadequate and rarely are they brought together within a common framework. This is a necessary task, however, given the range of conditions revealed in subsequent chapters on individual Healthy Cities Projects. A number of cities are already coming together to define joint approaches to measuring health and the components of a healthy city. The establishment of evaluation systems to support the development of effective policies which improve health and reduce inequalities would be a major contribution to achieving the vision of 'Health for All'.

References and further reading

Black Report (1980) *Inequalities in Health: Report of a Research Working Group*, London: Department of Health and Social Security.

Cheshire, P.C. and Hay, D.G. (1989) *Urban Problems in Western Europe: An Economic Analysis*, London: Unwin and Hyman.

Health Promotion: An International Journal (1988), 3(1) Oxford University Press. This issue is devoted entirely to health promotion indicators.

Seedhouse, D. (1986) *Health: The Foundations For Achievement*, Bristol: Wiley.

Thunhurst, C. (1985) *Poverty and Health in the City of Sheffield*, Health and Consumer Services Department, Sheffield City Council.

Townsend, P., Philhimore, P. and Beattie, A. (1986) *Inequalities in Health in the Northern Health Region*, Northern Regional Health Authority and the University of Bristol.

Whitehead, M. (1987) *The Health Divide: Inequalities in Health in the 1980's*, London: Health Education Council.

Urban health:
a global overview

The development of the Healthy Cities Project in Canada

Trevor Hancock

A perspective on Canada

Canada is a curious country, a strange hybrid of European and American values, of English and French culture, a vast country with a highly urbanized society. Most Canadians live in cities, and some 80–90 per cent live within 100 miles of the US border: Canada is in some respects a 5,000-mile long, 100-mile wide ribbon.

It has been said that while Americans are very sure of who and what they are, of their 'manifest destiny', Canadians are sure of what they are not – they are not Americans. Canada is the part of North America that did not have a revolution, but instead became the place of refuge for British loyalists fleeing from the American Revolution. Thus Canada remained a part of the British Empire, not becoming independent until 1867. This meant that Canada retained many of the British traditions, including a parliamentary system and a belief in good government.

Canada is said to have two 'founding nations', English and French, and is indeed an officially bilingual country. (Of course, this ignores the fact that when Canada was 'discovered' by Europeans, it already had a number of 'founding nations', the Native people – Indian and Inuit (Eskimo) – who have lived there for thousands of years.) And while Canadian culture has been heavily influenced by the American neighbours (to the extent that to Europeans Canadian lifestyle appears American) Canada is very distinct from the USA in its social values and systems and is in this respect closer in many ways to Europe.

One of the most obvious differences is that Canada has a strong belief in universal social benefits and a European-style welfare state. (Indeed, when US President Bush in his inaugural address in 1989 said he wanted 'a kinder, gentler nation', the joke going the rounds was that he had found it, and it's called Canada.) The most popular social programme of all is the national health insurance programme. While this was not introduced as early as many of the European programmes, by 1972 Canadians had universal health insurance.

And then a strange thing happened. Just at the time when the full power and might of the medical model had received the ultimate accolade of being given, in effect, a government-sanctioned monopoly on the health of Canadians, the government threw the whole concept into question.

A new perspective on the health of Canadians

In 1974 the Canadian Department of Health and Welfare quietly issued a report on the health of Canadians which would have a dramatic effect on health thinking – in the industrialized world especially – and would lead, indirectly, to the Healthy Cities movement. The report, titled *A New Perspective on the Health of Canadians* but more often called the Lalonde Report after the minister who issued it, began by accepting Professor Thomas McKeown's work, which indicated that, contrary to popular belief, the major factor in the improvement of health in the nineteenth and twentieth centuries was not medical care but a range of social and environmental changes. In particular, he pointed to economic growth, reduced family size, improved agriculture and food processing and distribution leading to improved nutrition, improved hygiene and sanitation, better living and working conditions and, only latterly, immunization and medical care. The Lalonde Report accepted this argument and applied it to today, concluding that major improvements in the health of Canadians would result primarily from changes in their lifestyle and their environment, and only secondarily from improvement in health care organization and medical services. The report also proposed several strategies, including the development of national health goals and suggested that health promotion was an important new priority; this led to the establishment in 1976 of the Health Promotion Directorate.

The Lalonde Report had an important effect on health thinking in both Europe and the USA in the 1970s, leading to the acceptance by government and academics of the need for a major rethinking of health and thus to the renaissance of the public health movement.

A municipal perspective on health

Some of that new thinking obviously rubbed off at other levels of government too, most notably at the local level in Toronto, where the seed that was to become the Healthy Cities movement was sown in 1978. Faced with a major discrepancy between the new environmental and social threats to health and a traditional and somewhat moribund public health department, the City of Toronto's Board of Health established a planning committee. Their 1978 report, *Public Health in the 1980's*, was in its way the Lalonde Report of municipal public health. It advocated a new approach to public health, emphasizing social and political action and community development to address the broad social and environmental threats to health. The report also placed a strong emphasis on good health status data, data-based planning, research and education, and a structural and functional reorganization of the public health department to emphasize team management, decentralization and community-based organization.

One of the most important consequences of the report was the establishment in 1979 of the Health Advocacy Unit, which became the cutting edge of the new public health in Toronto. This unit began to address itself to the fundamental principles of public health – ecological sanity and social justice – through reports and actions focusing on the relationships between poverty and health, the health effects of our 'chemical society' and the health complications of public policy. The unit also undertook a city-wide community health survey and data-based planning for health. Its pioneering work in the area of environmental health led in time to the establishment of the first municipal Environmental Protection Office in Canada, while its anti-smoking advocacy laid the groundwork for Canada's first municipal by-law regulating smoking in the work-place.

From Public Health to a Healthy City

This broad socio-ecological, policy-focused and community-orientated approach to public health led, perhaps inevitably, to a consideration of how to make Toronto a more healthy city; indeed the Department of Public Health in 1982 adopted as its mission statement 'to make Toronto the healthiest city in North America' (1988). And that, of course, posed a problem. Because it quickly became clear that the health of the city – or to be more precise, the health of the city's population – was the result of the actions of many groups other than the Department of Public Health, not only in city government, but in the business and voluntary sectors, in the community and in other levels of government.

So in 1984, as part of the events marking the centennial of the Board of Health, the Board hosted a workshop called 'Healthy Toronto 2000', which brought together a wide variety of sectors and interest groups to begin to explore how to make Toronto a more healthy city. One of the people in Toronto at the time was Ilona Kickbusch, Health Promotion Officer for the World Health Organization in Europe. She took the idea of a Healthy City back to Europe with her and the rest, as they say, is history – and another chapter in this book (see Chapter 19).

From Healthy Cities to Healthy Communities

While the Healthy City idea originated in Toronto, it was in Europe, under WHO's leadership, that the full potential of the concept was realized. But as the project grew in Europe, the importance of developing a Canadian version of the project became apparent. What emerged, however, is a very different and perhaps a very Canadian project.

The first unique aspect of the Canadian project concerns how it is managed and where it is housed. Canada has a strong tradition of non-governmental organizations playing an important role, especially in the public health sector. Thus, an obvious starting-point for the Canadian Healthy Cities project was the Canadian Public Health Association. However, the Association and the Health Promotion Directorate who funded the development of the project, recognized that, as had become apparent in Toronto, a healthy city was not the product of the public health sector alone. Two other key sectors were identified, namely urban planners and municipal politicians. Thus, their national associations – the Canadian Institute of Planners and the Federation of Canadian Municipalities – were sought out as partners. Moreover, it was also recognized that one of the important strategies for a successful Healthy City Project is to ensure that it is not simply a Health Department project; indeed, the belief is that it won't work unless the health sector 'gives it away'. This principle was carried over to the national level, and the three partner associations agreed that the project should be housed at the Canadian Institute of Planners, with a national steering committee drawn from all three associations, but with a majority of members from local municipalities representing all the major regions of Canada and a mix of health, planning and political expertise. This steering committee directs the work of the office, which has a full-time co-ordinator, a secretary and some consulting and 'marketing' funds, but not a lot.

A second unique characteristic of the Canadian project, and one that has created some controversy, is that it is called the Canadian Healthy *Communities* Project and it is open to all sizes of municipality, from a population of a couple of thousand to large cities. This change of title reflects the fact that, compared to Europe, there are only a few cities, or places that consider themselves cities, in Canada. The Federation of Municipalities was particularly emphatic in pointing out that calling the project 'Healthy Cities' would exclude a large proportion of their member municipalities. However, while the project is called 'Healthy Communities', the focus is still local government and joining the project ultimately requires a resolution to be passed by the council. As the project has developed, it has become clear that there are some real advantages to working with smaller municipalities. They benefit from a much more intimate local government, a smaller bureaucracy and closer links to their community. Creating intersectoral links and initiating change appears to be much easier and occurs much more rapidly in these smaller municipalities than in the larger cities such as Toronto.

A third unique aspect of the Canadian project is that it is open to any community that wants to join; there is no selection process. In part, this was a deliberate strategy to avoid creating a two-tier project, those selected to be 'in' the project and those left out, a status that might create problems between communities. Also, it was a recognition of the fact that while the European project could hold out the status of being recognized by WHO, as well as some expectation of expert resources, there was no obvious benefit, in terms of status or resources, from joining the Canadian project.

There was some concern at first that this might result in communities joining the project without serious intentions, but in fact the effect seems to be the opposite. Since there are no clear bonuses or incentives to joining the project, only those communities that are serious about it, who have something going on and want to share and to learn, can be bothered to join.

Another typically Canadian aspect of the Healthy Cities concept has been the emergence of parallel projects in other provinces, most notably in Quebec and British Columbia. In the province of Quebec, a Francophone project suited to the different culture and organization of Quebec's municipalities has been established by the Quebec Public Health Association, with links to other Francophone national networks. The Quebec project, known as 'Villes et Villages en Sante' is closely linked to the Canadian project, but has its own office and staff. The network of Quebecois healthy communities is the largest, best organized and most active in Canada. It is interesting to consider why this is so. In addition to the obvious energy and enthusiasm of the project co-ordinator and his staff, it is perhaps linked to the fact that in Quebec, in 1974, municipal public health was abolished and most of the public health responsibilities were transferred to regional health authorities (as happened in the UK at about the same time). Thus, local government lost its influence on the health conditions of its citizens, while public health lost its influence on the political decisions that affect health at the local level. Could it be that the healthy community concept provides both local governments and regional health authorities with the opportunity they both need to influence each other and to improve the public's health and quality of life?

Conclusion

The Canadian influence on the development of health promotion and the Healthy Cities concept has been considerable, though quite why this is so is hard to tell.

The Canadian Healthy Communities Project is distinct from the WHO project in three important respects:

1 It is jointly organized by three national associations and is run out of the offices of the national association of urban planners.
2 Its focus is not exclusively on 'cities' but all sizes of local governments.
3 It is open to any community that wishes to join.

The national project has been established for too short a time to evaluate it. However, it is clear that in Canada, as elsewhere, the Healthy City/ Community concept is an important one that seems to speak to the concerns of many different communities across the country and in both 'founding nations'. (There are also efforts underway to involve native communities in the project.) In that sense, the project is already a success. In terms of its ability to re-set the values underlying the decisions we make in planning and operating our communities, only time will tell.

References and further reading

Department of Public Health (1978) *Public Health in the 1980's*, Toronto: Board of Health.
Department of Public Health (1988) *Healthy Toronto 2000*, Toronto: Board of Health.
Evers, A., Farrant, W. and Trojan, A. (1990) *Local Healthy Public Policy*, Boulder, Colorado: Westview Press.
Hancock, T. (1982) 'Health as a Social and Political Issue: Toronto's Health Advocacy Unit', in D.P. Lumsden (ed.) *Community Mental Health Action*, Ottawa: Canadian Public Health Association.
Hancock, T. (1986) 'Beyond Lalonde: Looking Back at "A New Perspective on the Health of Canadians"', *Health Promotion* 1(1): 93–100.
Hancock, T. (1990) 'From "Public Health in the 1980's" to "Healthy Toronto 2000": The Development of Healthy Public Policy in Toronto', in A. Evers, W. Farrant and A. Trojan (eds) *Local Healthy Public Policy*, Boulder, Colorado: Westview Press.
Lalonde, M. (1974) *A New Perspective on the Health of Canadians*, Ottawa: Government of Canada.
McKeown, T. (1979) *The Role of Medicine – Dream, Mirage or Nemesis*, Princeton, NJ: Princeton University Press.
Szreter, S. (1988) 'The Importance of Social Intervention in Britain's Mortality Decline in 1850–1914: A Re-interpretation of the Role of Public Health', *Social History of Medicine* 1(1): 1–38.

Contact

Canadian Healthy Communities Project, 126 York Street, #404, Ottawa, Ontario, Canada K1N 5T5, Tel.: (613) 233-1617.

6

Healthy Cities in the United States

Beverly C. Flynn

Introduction

In order to analyse the Healthy Cities movement in the United States, an understanding of not only the history of the Healthy Cities movement but also the socio-political and public health environments of the United States is important. Much of what is occurring in Healthy Cities in the USA is a reflection of community-based health promotion programmes that have been supported at state and federal levels by private and/or public monies. Although the USA has a history of public and private funding for innovations that occur at the local level, public financing of local efforts has decreased over the last decade. Local communities must pick up the pieces of a fragmented system and address health issues without adequate public funding.

This chapter provides a brief analysis of a number of factors affecting the socio-political and public health environments in the USA and presents selected health promotion efforts as they relate to the Healthy Cities movement. Examples of Healthy City initiatives in the USA are provided with a discussion of some of their similarities and differences. The facilitators and barriers of Healthy Cities in the USA are discussed which suggest future issues that need to be resolved before the movement can be institutionalized at the local level.

Socio-political and public health environments

There is an increasing belief in the world today that people can take active steps that will improve their lives, which has been interpreted by some analysts that the world is moving towards democracy. In the United States there are a number of theories of democracy with as many competing views of what really drives the political scene. The USA has been called a nation of joiners and many believe that pluralism is the dominant explanatory theory. Pluralism is a form of democracy in which it is thought that the individual joins with others to achieve political goals (Dahl 1967). The interest or pressure group operates as a means of translating political goals from people to the legislature. In reality, pluralism is an imperfect form of representation as not all interest groups have equal resources or equal access to policy-makers. Because of this unequal distribution of political resources, the political process in the USA is subject to shifts with the group with the greatest power at the time being able to influence policy decisions the most.

The cut-back in federal funding for health in the USA during the 1980s has actually been an impetus to the Healthy Cities movement. One of the driving forces of the socio-political environment in the USA is decentraliza-tion, which impacts upon health by shifting the responsibility for health from federal to state and local levels without added financial resources. The tax bases on which state and local governments rely for funding public pro-grammes vary greatly with the result that the provision of programmes varies. Environments which promote healthy communities are not equally sought or attained. People at the local level realize that the inequalities in health persist. 'If we don't take charge of the health of our people, no one else will' has become a common attitude.

What is found in American society today is the fact that people feel they are more knowledgeable about current issues, perhaps as a result of the mass media, and people realize that they, too, can have an impact upon the decisions that affect their lives. These decisions, it is felt, are too important to be left in the hands of a few. These realizations are consistent with, and therefore supportive of, the Healthy Cities approach, which involves local participation in decisions affecting the health and quality of life in cities. However, in Healthy Cities one soon realizes that 'turfism', or protecting one's own 'piece of the pie', must be overcome for the benefit of the whole city. Healthy Cities has become a pathway for pluralism to work in promot-ing community health.

Health in the USA, not unlike other countries, has for a long time been seen as the responsibility of the medical profession leading Americans to seek 'quick fix' or curative approaches to health problems. Most of the health care dollar is spent on cures and treatment rather than on prevention of problems.

The responsibility for public health in the USA is at the local level with limited state funding for local programmes. The recent Institute of Medicine's (1988) report, *The Future of Public Health*, stated that 'public health is what we, as a society, do collectively to assure conditions in which people can be healthy' (1988: 1). Variations in public health programmes and services occur across states and communities. Public health in the USA was found to be in disarray, and a threat to the health of the public. The committee conducting this study found there was little consensus on the mission of public health, ranging from such services as indigent care, mental health, and environmental health in some agencies but not others. There was also a deficiency in public health expertise at the local level, particularly in the areas of public health management and epidemiology. The report also suggested that public health professionals failed to view politics as an essential element of their practice, not having built a constituency for public health, nor involving citizens in local public health decision-making, or continuing communications with elected officials about public health issues and solutions. As if these problems were not enough, public health professionals have an uneasy relationship with the medical profession which has not furthered the public's health.

If one would look at the history of public health in the USA, many of our distinguished leaders have been able to bring together sets of skills that provide examples to follow. Certainly, Lillian Wald, the first public health nurse, was able to use her technical knowledge and skill in providing direct services to people in their homes, to involve local citizens in decision-making at the Henry Street Settlement in New York City and, at the same time, to influence President Taft in 1912 to sign a Bill creating the US Children's Bureau. The Children's Bureau was formed to investigate and report on issues related to the welfare of children among all classes of people.

The recommendations of the Institute of Medicine's report reminds public health professionals of their rich heritage. These recommendations challenge local health departments to conduct community health assessments, to be more proactive in the health policy area, to seek co-operative and collaborative efforts instead of competitiveness, and to be responsible for filling the gaps in health care delivery under the rubric of the health department's responsibility to assure that basic services exist in the community. Clearly, Healthy Cities is one approach that provides an avenue in which to address many of these recommendations in the United States.

Health promotion in the USA

Health promotion efforts in the United States have existed over the course of American history and range from individual lifestyle change to a focus on community-based programmes. This section briefly presents selected current federal health promotion efforts that have implications for the Healthy Cities movement.

The Year 2000 Objectives build upon the 1990 Objectives (*Promoting Health/Preventing Disease* 1980) which were published following the report *Healthy People: The Surgeon General's Report on Health Promotion and Disease Prevention* (1979). The 1990 Objectives addressed improvements in health status, risk reduction, public and professional awareness, health services and protective measures, and surveillance and evaluation expressed in measurable targets. In 1986 an interim assessment of these objectives was published. Although they did well on most objectives, the citizens of the United States did not look very healthy in the areas of pregnancy and infant health, family planning, nutrition, fitness and exercise, and violent behaviour.

Although the Year 2000 Objectives are still under revision, more of these objectives are community-level targets. For example they address: per population community swimming pools, people trails, and park and recreation space; large city outreach programmes to contact drug abusers and deliver risk reduction messages; air quality; and local public information systems on hazardous chemicals.

Although considerably more extensive, these health objectives for the nation are much like the World Health Organization's (WHO) thirty-eight European targets being used by the European Healthy Cities Programme. In fact one of the aims of the United States Department of Health and Human Services (USDHHS) Office of Disease Prevention and Health Promotion, in promoting healthy communities in the USA, is to have the Health Objectives for the Year 2000 used by local communities (Files 1990).

Two other national initiatives are worth mentioning as they have elements of the Healthy Cities process. The first is Planned Approach to Community Health (PATCH), which was developed by the US Centers for Disease Control (CDC). PATCH has a mission to reduce the risk factors for the leading causes of preventable morbidity, mortality, disability and injury. This programme is designed to help communities plan, implement and evaluate health promotion and health education programmes. A local co-ordinator, a core group, and a community group are integral to the PATCH process. The local co-ordinator usually has responsibility for health education at a local health agency. The core group consists of at least three people who have a long-term commitment to PATCH and assists the local co-ordinator in the programme's administrative functions and in identifying resources to accomplish goals. The community group consists of private citizens, political office-holders, and individuals from service organizations and private companies. The community group participates in developing programme objectives and serves on working committees. Both the core and community groups assist in implementing programme activities. The state health department and CDC provide technical assistance and training to communities.

The second and more recent programme is called the Assessment Protocol for Excellence in Public Health (APEX/PH) (1989). The programme was initiated by the National Association of County Health Officials and is a collaborative effort with the American Public Health Association, the Association of Schools of Public Health, CDC, and the United States Conference of Local Health officers. APEX/PH is a self-assessment process for use by local health departments to assist them in meeting the community's health needs. A manual guides the assessment and improvement of the organization's capabilities, the assessment of the health status of the community, and the involvement of the community in pursuing public health objectives. Thirteen local health departments are currently involved as demonstration sites throughout the country. These demonstrations concluded in June 1990.

PATCH and APEX/PH have elements of the Healthy Cities process including community assessments and involving community people in local decisions about health promotion and public health. These programmes indicate a national concern with changing the way community health is being practised by opening the decision-making process to include the community itself.

Healthy Cities initiatives in the USA

Two Healthy Cities initiatives are underway in the United States. One, Healthy Cities Indiana (see Chapter 21), is a collaborative programme between the Indiana University School of Nursing, Indiana Public Health Association, and six Indiana cities, begun in August 1988 with a grant from the Kellogg Foundation. The second, the California Healthy Cities Project (see Chapter 20), is funded by the California State Department of Health Services and began selecting their cities in August 1989. Although both these initiatives are presented in Part IV, an analysis of similarities and differences between these two programmes may be useful here. Both Indiana and California are adapting the WHO European Healthy Cities model in their respective states. In the Indiana experience the programme directors and the Indiana Public Health Association targeted cities for participation in the programme and involved city leaders in a process of deciding whether or not there was enough local support to participate for at least three years. Once this decision was made the Mayor and local health officer signed a memorandum of understanding which indicated the policy implications of this decision for the city. The cities each decided to form a broad-based local Healthy City Committee – a public–private partnership – and to go through a process of assessing their city's health strengths and problems, establishing priorities, finding solutions and resources, and monitoring their successes and limitations in promoting healthy public policies. Technical support for each of the cities is provided by the Healthy Cities Indiana project directors and staff. Currently the National League of Cities is collaborating with the Healthy Cities Indiana Resource Center in the dissemination phase of the programme. Through the National League of Cities' network of elected officials from about 16,000 cities throughout the USA, Healthy Cities information and technical support is being provided.

In the California experience, a request for proposals from 450 cities was made by the project directors. Five initial cities and later two more were selected based on: commitment of city leadership and the passage of a city council resolution; broad community involvement by multiple sectors on a steering committee; and intervention strategies that were feasible, innovative, transferable and/or repeatable. Cities participate in the project one year at a time with an annual renewal application required (Twiss 1990).

In October 1989 the National Civic League entered a Collaborative Agreement with the USDHHS Office of Disease Prevention and Health Promotion to promote healthy communities in the United States. John Parr of the National Civic League hopes this programme will help communities understand the connection between community health, quality of life, and economic development (Parr 1990). The programme will provide information and advice on how to get a project started, and organize conferences and workshops on the healthy community concept. The National Civic League also proposes that a number of healthy community pilot projects be established across the nation (*Civic Action* 1990).

Ashley Files of the Office of Disease Prevention and Health Promotion indicated that her office was interested in promoting community-based health promotion rather than promoting one style of healthy cities. Files's Office wants to have communities look at health holistically and to use the National Health Objectives for the Year 2000. An emphasis will be given to measurable change through quantitative data, rather than to qualitative changes (Files 1990).

Two other significant efforts are related to the Healthy Cities movement in the USA. One is the KidsPlace project, which originated in Seattle, Washington. KidsPlace was jointly founded by the city of Seattle and two private organizations and aims to place children and their families high on the city's political, cultural and economic agenda. One of the first steps, taken in 1984, was a survey of Seattle's children and youth to determine what the city would be like if it were a healthy place for kids. Survey results led to the formation of a planning document, *The KidsPlace Action Agenda 1985–1990*, a Kids-Board of teenagers that lobbies City Hall on issues of concern to teens, an Annual KidsDay where all activities in the city are free to children ('KidsPlace: A Kids' Lobby for a Vital Seattle', Seattle, Washington, 1987). The KidsPlace process has been replicated in over twelve cities in North America, including Anchorage, Alaska to St Louis, Missouri.

The second programme has been cited by the National Civic League as one of the US Healthy Community Projects: the Colorado Action for Healthy People (CAHP) (*Civic Action* 1990). This project is in its third year of funding with support from the Colorado Trust, the Henry J. Kaiser Family Foundation and the Comprecare Foundation. CAHP helps communities initiate and expand their health promotion activities, offers technical assistance and seed money to local projects, and serves as a networking and resource centre. In working with a coalition of public and private community leaders interested in developing a health promotion project to prevent serious health risks, CAHP assists with community needs assessments.

Clearly from these Healthy City initiatives in the USA, there is no single Healthy Cities model that is emerging. Variations occur across programmes and projects, which is consistent with the history of health promotion in the USA.

The future of Healthy Cities in the USA

The socio-political and public health environments at the local levels are ripe for the expansion of Healthy Cities in the USA. It is clear from the presentations of the various Healthy City and related programmes that similar words are used but they have very different meanings across projects. The Healthy Cities movement in the USA is not being implemented uniformly in different parts of the country. In some areas, it is clearly a community development approach to community health and in others it is more project-specific using traditional approaches to planning.

An analysis of the various Healthy City projects and interviews with people responsible for Healthy City programmes in the United States suggests these major facilitators of the Healthy Cities movements:

1 As the responsibility for health shifts from federal to state and local levels, the already limited financial and other resources available to communities are further strained. Communities are challenged to address the increasingly complex problems that have health effects on their citizens. The Healthy Cities movement brings to the community an opportunity to approach problems with new resources through a private and public partnership which views the city holistically. All sectors are finding they need to transfer this holistic view of their city's health not only into the formation of broad-based city plans, but also into their own sector's action plans.
2 The environmental movement is gaining strength in the USA and, at the same time, people are seeing linkages between health, environment and economic development of communities. The very existence of the human race is deemed at risk if these broader health issues are not resolved. People are responding to this new recognition of risk by asking what the individual can do to ameliorate the danger. Healthy Cities provides an avenue in which people can respond.
3 As Healthy Cities and similar local initiatives increase, networks across cities and within cities are forming. These networks lead to an exchange of information and co-operation which is strengthening the Healthy Cities movement.

Some of the facilitators to the Healthy Cities movement in the United States are also barriers to the movement. For example, limited financial and other resources may be facilitators, but they are also barriers to local action. The limited resources available to localities means there is considerable competition for these scarce resources from other interests. Those interests that are better organized and have more skilful leaders may in fact succeed in drawing available resources away from investments in health. Healthy Cities may in fact provide a means for overcoming competing interests by demonstrating the commonalities of their opposing views, but it will not be an easy task.

An additional barrier that must be overcome in the United States is the debate over whether public health is a county function or a responsibility of the city. This debate is compounded by the difficulty which many citizens have in understanding the overlapping jurisdictions of county and city government. The size of the city also has been noted as a barrier, in that large cities are more complex and communication across various sectors may be more difficult.

Conclusion

The ultimate test of the success of Healthy Cities in the United States will be whether or not these programmes are sustainable over time and the extent to which inequalities in health are significantly addressed. The latter challenge, after all, continues regardless of country: Health for All as a means to social justice in society.

References and further reading

Civic Action (Jan.–Feb. 1990) Denver, Col: National Civic League.
Dahl, R. (1967) *Pluralist Democracy in the United States: Conflict and Consent*, Chicago, Ill: Rand McNally.
Files, A. (1990) Personal communication, 7 March.
Healthy People: The Surgeon General's Report of Health Promotion and Disease Prevention (1979) Washington, DC: US Department of Health and Human Services.
Institute of Medicine (1988) *The Future of Public Health*, Washington, DC: National Academy Press.
'KidsPlace: A Kids' Lobby for a Vital Seattle, Seattle, Washington' (1987) in J.E. Kyle (ed.) *Children, Families and Cities*, Washington, DC: National League of Cities, 13–16.
Parr, J. (1990) Personal communication, 12 March.
Planned Approach to Community Health (updated) Atlanta, Ga: US Center for Disease Control.
Promoting Health/Preventing Disease: Year 1990 Objectives for the Nation (1980) Washington, DC: US Department of Health and Human Services.
Promoting Health/Preventing Disease: Year 2000 Objectives for the Nation (1989) Washington, DC: US Department of Health and Human Services.
The APEX/PH Project: December 1989 Fact Sheet (1989) Washington, DC: National Association of County Health Officials.
The 1990 Health Objectives for the Nation: A Midcourse Review (1986) Washington, DC: US Department of Health and Human Services.
Twiss, J. (1990) Personal communication, 7 March.

7

Healthy Cities in Australia

Lewis Kaplan

The impetus for the Australian Healthy Cities Project came primarily through a number of personal contacts, notably a secondment of an officer from the Australian Federal Department of Community Services and Health to the Regional Office for Health Promotion in WHO Europe to assist with the preparations for the second international conference on Health Promotion, which was held in Adelaide in May 1988. Other Healthy Cities contacts with key players in the health promotion field in Australia arose through international conferences at a time when there was widespread excitement about the notion of the New Public Health taking over where health education and 'lifestyle' programmes left off.

The main Healthy Cities contacts made in Australia were with individuals associated with the Community Health movement, and it was almost inevitable that the Australian Community Health Association (ACHA) became the national auspice of the project. The ACHA is a federally funded non-government organization which was established in 1984 to promote and lobby for community health at the national level. The ACHA had a track record of running a difficult project in the form of the Community Health Accreditation and Standards Project, which was moving into gear in some states as well as at a national level at the time of the Healthy Cities initiative. There was a certain amount of doubt within ACHA about the wisdom of running a project like Healthy Cities with three autonomous pilot cities. It could well have proved to be impossible to administer effectively, but this did not turn out to be an insurmountable problem.

The level of interest in Healthy Cities in Europe exceeded all expectations. It had a parallel in Australia where there was a desire, following recommendations in the Better Health Commission's report and the Review of Community Health, both published in 1986, to establish a significant health

promotion project which had a major emphasis on intersectoral collaboration. Healthy Cities became that project – the largest project of the National
Health Promotion Programme, and thus of particular interest to politicians
and bureaucrats in terms of its potential for success, for community participation, local resourcing and regional replication.

The Healthy Cities Australia Pilot Project was funded in May 1987 by the
Federal Department of Community Services and Health. Funding came from
the National Health Promotion Programme and was channelled via the
national sponsor, the Australian Community Health Association (ACHA) to
the three pilot cities of Canberra (Australian Capital Territory – ACT), the
Illawarra (New South Wales) and Noarlunga (South Australia) and to the
national secretariat housed in the ACHA office. The three cities were chosen
in part because they were very different from each other and would thus
provide a broad range of models for other Australian communities. The
problems with the disparity between the pilot cities centred around data-
gathering and evaluation. How would each city be compared to the others?
In the event, cross-city health status comparisons were not seen to be an
appropriate indicator for the project in the Australian context.

Criteria and objectives

In Australia, the pilot project adapted seven criteria for city participation
from material supplied by the WHO European office. The first two criteria
for participation were to develop a political commitment to improving the
health of a city through the formation of a high-level intersectoral reference
group and a management committee comprising officers from various government and non-government agencies, complemented by community members
representing local organizations and even interested individuals. Subsequent
criteria reflected the project's commitment to reorienting services in favour of
the more disadvantaged in the community, to gathering data with a distinct
bias towards social health indicators, to active and strong relationships
between the pilot projects and the media, and between the pilot cities and any
other cities wishing to participate in the Healthy Cities movement.

The objectives of the pilot project as found in the original submission were
useful for establishing the project, but after one year of operation, it was
realized that they would be difficult to apply to an evaluation which it was
intended to conduct at the end of the three years. With this in mind, the
national and pilot city objectives were rewritten and the revised version
approved by the National Health Promotion Programme Secretariat half way
through the pilot project. Objectives for a project of this type are in any case
difficult to write, given that most of the activities associated with the project
were about process rather than outcome. A separate Research and Evaluation
subcommittee was established by the Project Executive to oversee the data-
gathering and analysis and evaluation processes, both to guide the pilot cities

and the national secretariat and to provide a level of consistency between the pilot cities.

Structures and functions

The Healthy Cities Australia Project was funded as a three-year national pilot. A submission was funded in May 1987 for three years for a total of A$654,900. This figure was made up of A$52,000 annually for each of the three pilot cities and A$62,300 annually for the national secretariat. The funds covered a project officer, part-time administrative support and a modest travel and communications budget for each pilot city and for the national secretariat.

The usual basis for major programmes of federal–state cost share was replaced with a commitment from partner sponsors in each of the pilot cities to match the federal funding with local resourcing. This was again a mirror of what was happening in Europe, where WHO for the first time was working directly with cities, bypassing the normal channels of member states' Ministries of Health. The Australian national secretariat was one of the first to be established. It has been followed by national secretariats in Canada, UK, France and Germany.

Over the three years of the project, the proportion of the ACHA national office which was given over to supporting the Healthy Cities Project increased significantly, while the financial arrangement did not alter. In the three pilot cities the principal partner sponsors were the area Health Services, but other organizations took an increasing role in resourcing the local activities of the pilot project.

In Canberra, ACT Community Services and Health (ACT CS&H – now Department of Health) provided the main local support in terms of office space, telephone and lending of staff and other facilities to allow the project to function and attract wider local support. Over the first year, the Healthy Cities Canberra project changed its official partner sponsor to the ACT Community Health Association (ACT CHA), an affiliate of the national ACHA. However, the Canberra Healthy Cities project retained its primary resource support from the ACT CS&H as the ACTCHA had no other liabilities or income. The Healthy Cities Project was the first project of the ACT CHA which did, however, provide most effective management and support.

The reason for the change of sponsor was largely bureaucratic in that the financial section of the ACT CS&H was not able to manage the extremely flexible demands of both project staff and the funding body, the National Health Promotion Programme. Once the financial function was accepted by the ACT CHA, financial reporting became the envy of the other two pilot cities, which were both sponsored by large partner organizations that took longer than was desirable to produce financial statements.

In the Illawarra a pair of partner sponsors emerged in the form of the School of Health Sciences at Wollongong University and the Illawarra Area Health Service. The local resourcing in the Illawarra included a senior officer seconded from the Health Service to work with the federally funded project officer. Offices were maintained in the University and at the Area Health Promotion Unit in town. This arrangement was fairly stable, and communication within the Illawarra project remained good throughout the three years. There was not always agreement about various policies and planned activities, but there was certainly a good level of discussion about them. In fact of the three pilot cities, the Illawarra showed most positive results for in-kind support for a variety of initiatives. Wollongong won the NSW award for most beautiful city for 1989 from the Keep Australia Beautiful Council in part because of the work of the Healthy Cities project.

The Noarlunga Healthy Cities Project has had the easiest time of the three pilot cities in terms of the level of local commitment and support from the start. There were always positive interactions between the project and the local sponsor partner, Noarlunga Health Services, which not only housed the project but also provided a high level of resource support as the project developed to the point of requiring funds additional to the agreed budget. There was also a strong relationship with the Southern Community Health Services Research Unit, an autonomous research establishment funded by the South Australian Health Commission. The Research Unit was able to assist with data collection and analysis as well as with the overall evaluation of local and national project activities.

Noarlunga did have a certain weakness in attracting local media support. However, this was structural rather than a result of any specific inability to arouse the media support which was a significant goal of the pilot project. When compared with the Illawarra and Canberra, it is immediately evident that the regional media of the latter two cities are geared to the same area that the project covers, whereas Noarlunga has to compete with the state capital, Adelaide for scarce media resources.

Practical achievements

One of the most common questions addressed to the project was 'What does Healthy Cities actually do?' In an attempt to answer this question a number of successful outcomes engendered by the project may be recorded.

In the Illawarra, for example, the local decision to clean up Lake Illawarra was co-ordinated by the Healthy Cities Project, with tremendous local response: over 2,500 volunteers, 220 local, state and national organizations together with resources estimated at over A$500,000 participated in 'Project Armada' over a wet and cold weekend in June 1989.

In Noarlunga, the Healthy Cities Project was able to bring conflicting groups to the negotiating table over the issue of clean water for the southern suburbs of Adelaide. Because of its relative neutrality, and because a wide range of different groups had a stake in the success of the Healthy Cities Project, previous conflict was replaced by co-operation. The state level authorities agreed to respond to local concerns about the quality of drinking water by investing in a water filtration plant as a commitment to the process of developing a Healthy Cities network.

In Canberra project staff and volunteers were able to put the New Public Health on to the political agenda when the ACT moved towards self-government and local politicians were keen to stand up and be counted in a city where health needs were largely perceived to be those of overdevelopment and health promotion and the new public health were acceptable strategies in a highly planned city with a centrally controlled bureaucracy.

These three examples are taken from dozens of smaller or larger 'successes' in which the Healthy Cities Projects have been involved. What is possibly more important from a global perspective is the emphasis throughout the Healthy Cities Project on reorientating thinking and planning processes away from curative medicine or even preventive medicine towards a broader and more positive definition of health. The project assisted many organizations and institutions at the local level to understand how they can and should have a much more active role in maintaining and promoting the 'Public Health'. This was exemplified in the Illawarra where a local 'Public Health Charter' was developed by the Project and signed at the end of 1989 by some thirty different organizations, most of which, through involvement on the Steering Committee of the Healthy Cities Project, had come to have a much clearer appreciation of the WHO definition of health and of their involvement in creating and maintaining it.

The other area in which the Healthy Cities Project may be said to have played a unique role is in the development of a truly intersectoral management structure. In order to achieve this, the project has had to retain a level of neutrality which is not conducive to the development of a significant bureaucratic power base. However, there had always been a commitment by project holders to Healthy Cities as a concept and a movement rather than as a parallel bureaucratic structure. Only in this way would local government Councils be prepared to accept and participate in Healthy Cities activities without the inevitable response of 'Don't expect us to fund this project once the pilot grant is finished.'

One area of less than desired success was the level of commitment by general 'members of the community' to active participation in the planning and management of the pilot project. Although this is not a new complaint, it was one that was voiced repeatedly in the pilot cities in as much as the project was strongly predicated on the five action strands of the Ottawa Charter for Health Promotion (WHO 1986), which make particular reference to 'strengthening community action' and 'developing personal skills'.

One of the most interesting developments of the Healthy Cities Project was the involvement of an Aboriginal community health service, Nganampa Health Council, which is run by the Anangu Pitjatjantjara people in northern South Australia. When the original proposal for funding was submitted, one of the objectives was to include an Aboriginal community in the pilot project. The aim was to show that the intersectoral nature of Healthy Cities, together with the emphasis on a broad definition of health and social health indicators, was equally applicable in a scattered rural community and in a complex urban environment.

Unfortunately, the funding body was not prepared to accept the inclusion of a fourth pilot city with very different parameters from the original three. There was widespread support for the inclusion of the Nganampa Health Council – from the Federal Minister for Aboriginal Affairs, the South Australian Health Commission as well as from other peak Aboriginal organizations in the health sector. The funding for Nganampa eventually came from the Australian Freedom from Hunger Campaign and was subsequently matched by the South Australian Health Commission's Social Justice Strategy. The irony was that the Nganampa Health Council was better placed to achieve the project's objectives than were the three pilot cities at the time the project was started.

Where to from here?

The Healthy Cities Project in Australia has engendered a degree of national interest well beyond its limited capacity as a pilot project with little funding for promotional activities outside the pilot cities. The initial submission for funding included three national workshops each year to allow project holders to meet to learn from one another and report back to a wider audience. These workshops were initially small, but grew to an unexpected size with the seventh national workshop in Canberra hosting over 100 participants from every state and territory in the country. The project rapidly became more widely known through the dissemination of information kits, public speaking and a certain level of media exposure as well as by word of mouth in the health promotion and local government communities. It soon became apparent that a number of cities were already working towards the objectives embraced by the Healthy Cities Project, or were ready to adopt some or all of the criteria for participation promoted by the project.

Over the three years of the pilot project more than thirty cities expressed an active interest in joining the proposed national network. The level of interest varied widely from an information exchange with interested community development workers to cities which took on a full commitment to the project with regular project committee meetings serviced by a project officer.

The national project organized a major conference called 'Healthy Cities Australia – Making the Connections: People, Communities and the Environment', held in Wollongong after almost three years of operation. Over two hundred delegates attended the conference at which the national network was launched. The timing of the conference was fortuitous as it came shortly before a federal election. A proposal for funding for a continuing national secretariat had been submitted to the new National Better Health Programme in December 1989, and an announcement of the funding was made at the conference on 12 February 1990. The National Secretariat would be continued for a further two years. However, it was made clear that there would be no further federal support for local initiatives beyond the three years in the pilot cities. This did not impede fifteen cities from making a commitment at the national conference to joining the national network. It is expected that the new enlarged secretariat will be able to work with another two dozen or so cities, towns and communities across Australia over the next two years to develop and refine the work achieved to date.

Reference

WHO (World Health Organization), Health and Welfare Canada, Canadian Public Health Association (1986) *Ottawa Charter for Health Promotion*, Copenhagen: WHO.

8

The emergence of urban health policy in developing countries

Trudy Harpham

Introduction: the problems become apparent

> The urban poor are at the interface between underdevelopment and industrialization and their disease patterns reflect the problems of both. From the first they carry a heavy burden of infectious diseases and malnutrition, while from the second they suffer the typical spectrum of chronic and social diseases.
>
> (Rossi-Espagnet 1984)

When Rossi-Espagnet stated that the urban poor in developing countries suffer the 'worst of both worlds' with regards to health problems there was relatively little research on which to base his claim. Since his seminal publication in 1984 there has been a proliferation of studies and articles which both highlight the rapid growth of poor urban communities in developing countries and describe their health problems. There has also been a shift in international, and in some cases, national organizations' perceptions of the problems. In the early 1980s, for example, the vision of primary health care in developing countries was distinctly rural. Urban areas were perceived as a homogeneous mass – an over-served elite absorbing far too much of the national health budget. Gradually the inequalities within urban areas are being realized and the growing enormity of the problem documented. International agencies now actively promote urban primary health care, for example, UNICEF and WHO. Bilateral agencies are beginning to fund urban primary health care (such as the Overseas Development Administration, UK). Non-governmental organizations (NGOs) have long been in the arena experimenting with small-scale pilot projects (see Harpham *et al.* 1988 for a review of these projects).

However, the development of urban primary health care is still at an early stage and this is one of the reasons why few national governments have yet committed themselves to an urban primary health policy. Questions remain such as: How transferable is the rural model of primary health care to the urban context? What particular constraints are there in poor urban communities? How does urban primary health care fit in with other programmes directed towards the urban poor? The objective of this chapter is to begin to attempt to answer these questions. The full answers will not be available before the mid-1990s when current large-scale urban health projects will be evaluated. However, there is now sufficient experience for us to stop describing the problem and to start discussing what can be done about it.

Identifying constraints and potential solutions

Many projects which have begun to implement primary health care (PHC) in poor urban communities in developing countries have experienced common problems. A summary of a selection of these problems is presented in Table 8.1. Many of these problems, or constraints, are characteristics of an urban environment and would not arise in a rural context in developing countries. For example, the dependence upon hospital services; the dependence upon a cash economy, the lack of land on which to grow food.

Some of the potential solutions are also unique to the urban environment emphasizing that working with urban communities presents unique opportunities in addition to problems. An example of this is the existence of the municipality (or local government). Local governments are generally more sensitive to community pressures and more open to community participation than development authorities or national ministries. Given the innovative nature of urban primary health care and common staff shortages at local levels there is occasionally a tendency to place implementation responsibility with national or provincial governments. However, local governments have a direct responsibility for local infrastructure development and hence provide a broad base for programme financing. In the long term it is often advantageous for the local government to be the implementing authority. This may provide more flexibility as national ministry of health norms for primary health care (often developed for rural programmes and therefore inappropriate) may not constrain a municipality's activities.

Slum upgrading

'Slum upgrading' is usually interpreted as the improvement of existing substandard housing in slums. Skinner *et al.*'s (1987) comprehensive review of slum upgrading points out that other inputs such as improved sanitation, water supply, drainage, paving and electricity are often part of upgrading projects. A common objective is to 'link' houses to an improved physical

Table 8.1   Constraints to environmental health improvements and the provision of community health services in poor urban areas of developing countries

Constraints	Potential solutions
1 Established dependence on curative service (e.g. private practitioners and hospitals) makes it difficult for PHC to achieve credibility.	Begin project with affordable, accessible curative services; add preventive activities gradually. Focus on rationalizing referral system.
2 Heterogeneous groups make definition of 'community' difficult.	Social analysis of neighbourhoods before defining 'communities'.
3 Greatest perceived need often security of tenure and improvements to housing.	Obtaining security of tenure as priority. Self-help housing schemes complement environmental health improvements.
4 Dependence on cash economy so difficult to pay CHWs (Community Health Workers) 'in kind' as often occurs in rural areas.	True volunteer CHWs or avoid CHWs or municipality employs the CHWs. The trend is towards the latter.
5 Little land on which to grow food to improve diet/nutritional status.	Income generation through skills training, facilitating low-cost loans.
6 Difficulty of co-ordinating sectors.	Use the municipality as umbrella organization; form an urban community development department within municipality.
7 Co-ordinating small-scale NGO activities difficult.	Form health co-ordinating committees at community and/or municipal levels.
8 Maintenance of physical assets (e.g. roads) difficult.	Form maintenance agreements between community and municipality.

infrastructure in order to stimulate improvements of the housing unit. These house improvements may be on a 'self-help' basis or government assisted. Most slum upgrading projects also aim to provide security of tenure. Although some of the inputs to a slum upgrading project may improve environmental health there have been few attempts to improve community health services in such projects until recently. Now, slum upgrading (focusing upon shelter) is extending to an integrated slum upgrading or 'slum improvement' which implies development in several sectors including health, education and income generation. Examples of this relatively new approach are the slum improvement projects in three Indian cities which the British Overseas Development Administration (UK) is assisting.

Indian urban health and the slum improvement projects

India is rapidly urbanizing. With an estimated 27 per cent of its population now living in urban areas and with some of the largest slums in Asia the central government of India is turning its attention to urban primary health care. In the mid-1980s the government established a high-level committee to recommend an approach towards urban primary health care. One of the main recommendations of this committee was that a health post should be established in each slum. The strength of medical, para-medical, non-medical staff and voluntary health workers (to be selected from the community) was to depend upon the population of the area. For example, for an area with a population below 5,000 there would be one nurse-midwife and two VHWs. However, the response of state authorities to these recommendations was luke-warm. One of the main mistakes of the committee was that they addressed only infrastructure strengthening and failed to consider other essential components of an effective health system like training, supervision, monitoring, evaluation, supply logistics and information, education and communication activities. Like numerous other health projects in developing countries 'support and supervision' was not anticipated or planned.

How far were these recommendations implemented? By the end of 1986 the number of health posts established in 127 different cities and towns was only 539 as against the target of 2,011. This situation led to the government rethinking and revised proposals are currently being developed for scores of cities in India. However, the approach is still firmly lodged within the health sector only.

In the mean time an alternative model has emerged. This is the model of integrated (multisectoral) slum improvement projects. The notable characteristics of the slum improvement projects in Hyderabad, Visakhapatnam and Indore (with Calcutta Municipality and Vijayawada possible additions in the future) are listed below:

1 They aim at total coverage of the slums in the city (180,000–460,000 beneficiaries).
2 They are implemented by the Community Development Departments of Municipalities or the City Development Authority, which have engineers, health and social workers.
3 They provide security of tenure to households in slums located on safe ground away from flooding or roads (this requires purchase of private land or transfer of government land). Land title (*patta*) is given to the head woman of the household.
4 Physical improvements account for about two-thirds of the total budget.
5 They are time-bound projects, typically four years' duration. The sustainability of recurrent costs is agreed between the community and the municipality. There is no attempt at cost-recovery in the initial project.
6 The typical cost is 441 rupees per capita over the duration of the project (1988 prices).

Within the 'health component' all the projects have community health workers (CHWs) who are selected from the community by the community council. They work for about four hours a day and are paid a small honorarium. They tend to be literate females of a wide age range. The CHWs create a family health folder for each household in the community which provides baseline data. The folders are maintained at the multifunctional community hall (built under the project) where a part-time auxiliary nurse-midwife and a doctor hold a clinic for four hours a day. The constitution of activities varies slightly between the projects but may include: child immunization, child growth monitoring, targeted supplementary feeding, family planning, antenatal and postnatal care, health education, promotion of oral rehydration therapy, identification, treatment and rehabilitation of disabled children, and treatment of minor ailments.

The health component is planned in conjunction with the other components of the project: physical upgrading and community development. So, for example, the installation of latrines or communal taps by engineers will coincide with health education on personal hygiene. The pre-school teacher will encourage pregnant mothers of her schoolchildren to attend antenatal checks in the community hall based clinic. Not everything is going as planned. Some of the problems currently faced are as follows:

1 Community health workers can spend too much time on over-elaborate monitoring forms.
2 Nurse-midwives are used as handmaidens of the doctors and are not undertaking their own, independent activities.
3 Referral system is often weak with no follow-up of referred patients.

Although the above projects are not yet complete they have already highlighted lessons which may apply to other health projects in poor urban communities in developing countries. The main lesson is that an integrated, multisectoral approach is appropriate. However, this approach creates extra strains upon management and field workers and intensive initial training and in-service training is required to ensure co-ordination between the wide range of activities. Although the projects are multisectoral the community development component should lead. No engineering or health services are introduced into communities before community organizers have explained the project, helped finalize the design and timing of inputs, stimulated formation of a neighbourhood committee and obtained baseline data. Post-project maintenance is considered at the earliest stage with agreements drawn up between the municipality and each community outlining a division of maintenance responsibilities (e.g. the community will replace electric light bulbs in the community hall where clinics and pre-schools are held, the municipality will collect garbage from skips twice a week).

In conclusion, urban primary health care is now on the agenda of several international, governmental and non-governmental agencies. Innovative projects are 'learning by doing'. There is a need to document these experiences in order to undertake comparative analyses of approaches and to develop appropriate urban health policy. Although policy needs to be tailored to individual countries and cities, experience so far suggests that the urban poor across countries have many common needs and common health problems.

The Indian slum improvement projects provide one model of action. We need more.

References and further reading

Harpham, T., Lusty, T. and Vaughan, P. (1988) *In the Shadow of the City: Community Health and the Urban Poor*, Oxford: Oxford University Press.
Rossi-Espagnet, A. (1984) *Primary Health Care in Urban Areas: Reaching the Urban Poor in Developing Countries*, A state of the art report by UNICEF and WHO, Report 2499M, Geneva: World Health Organization.
Skinner, R.J., Taylor, J. and Wegelin, E. (1987) *Shelter Upgrading for the Urban Poor: Evaluation of Third World Experience*, Manila: Island Publishing House.
UNICEF (1987) *Urban Primary Health Care: A Response to the Crisis or Urban Poverty*, Bangkok: UNICEF East Asia and Pakistan Regional Office.
WHO (1988a) *Improving Urban Health: A Programme for Action*, Report WHO/SHS/NHP/88.2, Geneva: World Health Organization.
WHO (1988b) *Urbanization and its Implications for Child Health: Potential for Action*, Geneva: World Health Organization.

9

Healthy Cities in developing countries

Marilyn Rice and Elizabeth Rasmusson

To begin to understand the major differences between developed and developing countries, it is important to note that for all the countries of the world, while the developing ones have 75 per cent of the world's population, they have only 17 per cent of the world's gross national product, 5 per cent of science and technology, 15 per cent of energy consumption, 30 per cent of the food grains, 11 per cent of the education spending, 18 per cent of export earnings, 8 per cent of industry, and 6 per cent of the health expenditure.

Between 1981 and 1986 the world economy, and particularly the developing market economies as a whole, experienced the most severe and prolonged recession since the 1930s. While most countries in South and East Asia managed to maintain satisfactory rates of growth over the period, 70 per cent of countries in Africa, the Middle East, and Latin America experienced negative cumulative growth rates in gross domestic product (GDP) per capita. There is widespread and growing evidence that in the early 1980s these economic changes, compounded in some areas, especially in Africa, by adverse climatic conditions, triggered a sharp reversal in the trend towards improvement in health, nutrition and education. Deterioration in child welfare has been documented in at least eight countries in Latin America, sixteen in Sub-Saharan Africa, three in North Africa and the Middle East, and four in South and East Asia. In many more countries, social progress has been negligible or slowed considerably (Cornia, Jolly and Stewart 1989). To a large degree, the extent to which the economic crisis affects people's health is very much determined by how governments respond to the crisis by trying to protect health and favour the most vulnerable groups of their populations (Musgrove 1987).

Certain infectious diseases show signs of new gains as a result of increasing poverty and an inability to meet people's basic needs. Every day, the number of children that die in India is greater than the total number of people who died in the Bhopal chemical disaster (when at least 2,000 people died in December 1984). Malnutrition remains a serious obstacle to health and to the development of human resources. A woman is more than 150 times more likely to die in childbirth in the developing world than in the developed world. If present trends continue, it will be impossible for the World Health Organization (WHO) to reach its goal of 'Health for All' by the year 2000 (HFA/2000) (Brundtland 1990).

Traditionally, health has been seen in isolation from other environmental factors that affect a person's health status, and the main 'solution' has been a medical one, that of providing mostly medical services and health education, both in a top-down, non-participative fashion. These two channels were thought to be a panacea for all health-related problems. However, evidence is growing of a strong relationship between health and the environment. Today there is widespread recognition that there are generic national and inter-national concerns that ultimately affect the health and well-being of the population. These concerns include medical waste disposal, radioactive and toxic wastes control, transportation, accidents, urbanization and automotive traffic, occupational health and safety, air and water pollution, acid rain, the greenhouse effect, and depletion of the planet's ozone layer. As the United Nations World Commission on Environment and Development has pointed out, developing countries face not only the public health problems that the industrialized world confronts, such as air pollution, poor water quality, solid waste disposal, and finding a balance between the economic incentives of development and a decent quality of life, but also many of the problems that richer countries have already overcome, such as a lack of adequate and safe water and sanitation facilities. At the same time, they must deal with the impacts on health of rapid and large-scale industrialization, urbanization, and technological development. The massive population growth makes it even more difficult to solve this double load of problems which outstrips the countries' economic development, retards their social development, and makes crushing demands on services, resources and the bearing capacity of the increasingly fragile environment (Kreisel 1990).

Innovations in medical science have had a profound effect on health and longevity. As a result, many children who previously would have died are now surviving. People are living much longer at the opposite end of the age spectrum as well. The sheer enormity of the population explosion cannot help but impress itself on the mind of anyone looking towards the future of the planet. Additionally, there are increasing numbers of people that are economically nonproductive (the very young, the very old, the disabled, the unemployed). As far back as 1965, the World Health Assembly provided the mandate to the World Health Organization to investigate more thoroughly the health aspects of population dynamics, human reproduction and family planning, stressing the intersectoral nature of population problems. In 1987, demographers placed the global human population at 5 billion. Unlike in times past, it did not take the population 100 years to double; rather the population size went from 2.5 billion to 5 billion in just thirty-seven years. This was a short enough time-span for people to see and remember this type of growth. China reached a level of 1 billion people and was faced with the problem of feeding, housing and clothing all of its citizens. It responded by setting a limit of one child per family policy and it has been accused of enforcing this family size restriction too vigorously. Bangladesh, with 107 million people, has instituted a two-child family policy and it will double its population in twenty-six years. Kenya, with 4 per cent growth rate and a population of 22 million is expected to double its population in eighteen years (Baldi 1988). In 1950 there were only two cities with a population over 10 million, New York and Paris. By 1975 that number had grown to seven. By the year 2000 over half of the people in the world will be living in cities and the number of cities over 10 million will be twenty-six. If we add the cities of the world with 5 million inhabitants, the number will be fifty-eight. In Latin America alone, 69 per cent of the population was living in urban centres in 1985, and it is projected that by the year 2025 up to 84 per cent of the population will be living in urban settings (United Nations 1986). The implications of these demographic projections for countries already struggling to promote economic and social development is staggering. Current projections indicate that if all goes well, global population will stabilize at 10.2 billion people somewhere between the year 2030 and 2070; 90 per cent of that growth will take place in the developing world.

With rapid urbanization, many new problems arise. Accidents, murder, suicide, alcohol and drug abuse, depression, widespread infections such as sexually transmitted disease (STD) and AIDS, as well as the increased problems of deteriorating infrastructures, increased immigration bringing new beliefs and cultures, and a breakdown in family structure and support systems which traditionally helped to sustain the way people worked and lived. Studies in Nicaragua, for example, indicate that whatever health benefits rural populations gained by moving to the city were overshadowed by the problems of overcrowding and pollution (Adegbola 1987). The magnitude of the health problems of the urban poor is rarely reflected in city health statistics. In spite of this, it is not surprising that infant mortality among the urban poor is often markedly higher than in rural areas (Lopez 1987). What infrastructures and services do exist, are stretched way beyond their capacity to offer any kind of quality, and they are limited to aiding only certain segments of the population, and often not those that are of highest risk and greatest need.

The relationship between housing and health is both intimate and complex. It is compounded by a large number of factors such as poverty, nutrition, levels of income and literacy. WHO estimates that 5 million of all annual deaths world-wide (10 per cent) could be prevented if all housing conditions met safe standard levels. WHO also estimated that an additional 2 million to 3 million cases of permanent disability could be prevented through improved housing. Many deficiencies in housing also adversely affect the residents' mental health (UNCHS 1988a).

Analysis of recent activities led to the conclusion that despite government efforts, the poor have done immeasurably more for themselves than governments have been able to do for them. The scale of the problems faced in Third World cities and initial governmental attitudes and resources allocated to address them have precluded major advances (UNCHS 1988a). Although governments may wish to contribute a great deal through formal programmes in the future, the persistent resource constraints are likely to make this increasingly difficult (UNCHS 1988a).

Conceptual framework for healthy communities

Clearly the task of working in urban centres in the developing world brings challenges and problems that the developed world on the one hand already has resolved and on the other hand has yet to face. The solutions, in turn, may sound very different, but in fact there are many similarities. In the Americas, the approach to Healthy Cities has been strongly linked to countries' efforts to concentrate on the decentralization of health and related services, and the strengthening of those services at the local level. As a dynamic part of its health education and health promotion activities, the Pan American Health Organization (PAHO) has called the new initiative 'Healthy Communities'. The focus on communities, rather than on cities *per se*, is due to the exploding demographic situation described above. In the large metropolises, participation in health activities is not carried out through full city co-operation, but rather neighbourhood by neighbourhood. These communities within communities often have their own specific needs, problems and potential resources. The initiative focuses on strengthening community participation and intersectoral collaboration in the development of local systems supportive of health. Implicit in this approach is an increased attention paid to social behaviours, placing more emphasis on actions of groups and organizations instead of looking at individual behaviours in isolation. Along with this focus is the need to reorientate factors that affect implementation such as national and local policies, allocation of resources and personnel, definition of priorities and issues, identification of viable solutions and activities to improve local conditions affecting health, and monitoring and evaluating initiatives in a continuing way to provide for effective reprogramming.

Institutions must expand their concept of health indicators to include social and environmental conditions, as well as individual and collective behaviours. It also means that there is a need to develop indicators of the types of services provided by the formal institutions and groups that go beyond the traditional ones of medical care, and include those of progress in promoting health and healthy social and environmental conditions. Institutions must look at their own capacity for providing for health promotion type services, and examine how they can play an appropriate role in these efforts.

This social approach to promoting health requires co-ordination and collaboration with many other sectors, groups and the community at large. Since the factors that affect the population's health include social, economic, cultural, political and infrastructure arenas, only through comprehensive efforts can realistic change come about. These efforts must begin with deliberation over problems and situations within communities, with participation on the part of all appropriate parties, including leaders that represent local government and policy, leaders of local institutions, organizations and groups, formal and informal community leaders, and members of the interested public. Through participatory planning these parties come to an agreement about which health promotion priorities they will start with, what strategies will be utilized, what specific actions will be taken and by whom, and what resources and personnel will be mobilized to achieve the desired outcomes. The process is one of continual negotiation, in which new strategies and activities can be added and old ones deleted as the needs change. The most important part of this approach is that the decision-making process is participatory and that responsibility for what is accomplished is assumed by the players involved. The essence of what makes this process function is the development and strengthening of partnerships and coalitions.

As a result of this type of participatory planning through partnerships, it is expected that all those involved will come to a new understanding of what primary health care is and how it applies at the community level. It requires collecting existing and new data and information from many different sources and sectors. So much of the needed information is already available, the difficult part is identifying where to get it and selecting what is most pertinent and appropriate. One of the outcomes of this type of assessment is the identification of all types of local inequities and pockets of populations with greatest need. This information needs to be made widely available in the community so that all people are able to discuss what needs to be done to improve health. It also highlights the health impact of existing policies and programmes, and the need to form new coalitions to eliminate the inequities and strengthen local ways of resolving local problems. From the political perspective, it places health in the centre of the public's debate about how to improve quality of life and how to create more choices for healthier lifestyles. Community leaders are identified to speak out for better health.

One of the most important outcomes of this problem-solving process is a greater self-reliance and improved power of advocacy and catalysing initiative for the community, which facilitates improvement of local social and environmental conditions, and in turn helps to create better quality of life and more equitable accessibility to services. A specific plan is developed to collect and distribute needed information about health, develop stronger intersectoral co-operation and provide adequate resources for health. This does not mean that service delivery organizations have less responsibility. On the contrary, they have a greater responsibility to be responsive to the requests and demands of the population they are supposed to serve, and to do so in a timely, appropriate and effective manner.

Developing world examples of Healthy Cities initiatives

Housing

A main objective of new governmental strategies in housing is one of creating conditions that enable self-help and mutual aid. Government support is provided for locally determined, self-organized, and self-managed settlement programmes based on individual and collective private initiatives. Specific examples of these enabling actions include: fostering community participation, increasing basic services, increasing availability of finance to the poor, increasing the supply of building materials, increasing land supply, strengthening urban management, and promoting training and education.

Rio de Janeiro's Favela do Gato, or 'Shanty Town of the Cats', provides an example of a peripheral urban community which has successfully organized and advocated the improvement of its housing conditions. Favela de Gato, like so many other urban areas in the Third World, grew up on Rio's periphery as rural residents left their homes, fleeing to the city in search of a better life. These men, women and children scavenged for wood, metal, cardboard or whatever materials they could find, to build their homes.

With the support of the Group for Community Projects of the University Federal Fluminese, the slum-dwellers negotiated with the national housing authority, which resulted in setting up seventy-one model houses and a community centre, granting of individual financing, and absorption by the public authorities of the costs for the land and infrastructure. Each family chose its site and the position of the house upon its plot of land, an unusual opportunity for a low-income housing scheme. The layout of a section of the favela was planned on the basis of the residents' wishes (Canedo, Elisa and Bienenstein 1985).

The housing plight of the urban poor in Latin America is not confined to the well-known slums and shanty towns encircling many large cities. Squalid, decaying buildings near the heart of the city are home also for many residents in such cities as São Paulo, Lima, Mexico City, and Santiago. Many of these tenements are former hotels and homes which have fallen into disrepair and have been abandoned. Although they have long since deteriorated, the buildings sometimes form an essential part of the historical patrimony of these cities; for this reason they have not been torn down, and it is unlikely that they will be (Welna 1988).

During Argentina's former military government, many of the urban poor left Buenos Aires when bulldozers stripped the city of its shanty towns in the late 1970s. However, many other residents remained close to the income sources and urban services found in the city. Since adequate housing is expensive and scarce, large numbers of those who stayed have taken up residence in the decaying buildings near the heart of the city. These overcrowded tenements are often structurally unsafe and provide no proper place to bathe, few, if any latrines, and limited or non-existent kitchen facilities.

Specifically, three types of housing are commonly available to Buenos Aires' inner-city poor. The first are decaying mansions on the south side of the city. These homes were divided into single-room tenements for European immigrants a century ago when their wealthy occupants moved to the northern neighbourhoods of the city. Another type of residence is the 'family hotel', or boarding house, where rooms are rented by the week with no contractual obligations on either side. A third housing option is to occupy vacant and decaying buildings illegally. All three types of dwellings often provide residents with unsafe and substandard housing.

Fortunately, efforts are being made by various groups to improve these conditions and provide better housing options for residents. Tenants' groups in Buenos Aires have devised two strategies for helping poor urban tenants renovate their homes. One plan provides technical assistance from university engineering students through the auspices of 'Grupo Habitat', an advisory organization that works with tenant groups. The other plan is to form a labour pool of tenants with construction skills who are available to make home improvements. The organization is also working to propose corrective legislation to change the difficult requirements involved in renting, and to reduce entrance costs for long-term apartments. The large initial costs, rather than the monthly payments, are what often exclude potential residents from renting.

'Grupo Habitat' has also devised a project that would transform tenant hotels into consortiums that could be managed by the tenants themselves. Hopefully the tenants could then undertake the physical improvements most of the hotels need, using part of their rental payments to finance the renovations. This could also prove appealing to hotel owners, since many owners pay wages to managers who have no personal interest in maintaining or improving the property (Welna 1988).

In some cities, slums which once sprawled throughout the downtown area are being encroached upon by developers wishing to expand. For most residents this has meant eviction. However, some residents in Bangkok have devised a creative scheme for solving this apparent impasse. Like thousands of other slum-dwellers in Thailand's capital city, the people of the Sengki neighbourhood faced eviction when real estate developers sought the land on which they lived. After a fire swept through the neighbourhood, owners cancelled leases, turning residents into squatters.

The condition of Sengki residents is not unique for Bangkok – of the more than one thousand slum communities in the city, over two hundred were threatened with eviction in 1988. Rehousing residents in a new area is a costly solution for the government and developers, and it is not even acceptable to many residents. Rather than move from their neighbourhood, residents of Sengki have developed an arrangement called 'land-sharing'. This system divides the slum into two parts, one for the landowner to develop as he wishes, the other is leased or sold to residents who organize themselves into a co-operative to build new homes. Landowners experience immediate financial gain and avoid long costly confrontations with tenants, while tenants gain small, but secure plots of land for their homes.

In the Sengki neighbourhood, a commercial loan was obtained by the neighbourhood housing co-operative for a down payment on part of the land. This land was then sold to residents at less than half of its market value. Owners will now be able to build new homes on their plots, choosing from various models which have been proposed to them, or building whatever type of home they wish. Residents' involvement in their neighbourhood will be encouraged through an election process, after which much of the administration will be given to the community itself. Support for the project came from the United Nations Development Programme and the UN Centre for Human Settlements (Habitat). Both of these organizations see land-sharing as a model for future slum clearing. At present, five other land-sharing projects in Bangkok are in various stages of completion (Jensen 1989).

Other problems/issues being addressed by Healthy Cities initiatives

Efforts by city-dwellers in the developing world to improve their quality of life have not been limited to issues of land tenure and housing. Communities have organized to work for a wide variety of shared goals ranging from improved sanitation to environmental education. These goals have been carried out under the auspices of the World Health Organization's Healthy Cities initiative, as well as through independent efforts.

La Paz, Bolivia has been the first Latin American city officially to embrace the WHO Healthy Cities initiative *per se*. In June 1989 a National Seminar was held in La Paz to introduce participants to the concepts of health promotion and Healthy Cities. Participants worked to define their goals and objectives, and by the end of the Conference they had developed an intersectoral 'Healthy City' plan for La Paz.

The plan is comprehensive and ambitious, introducing a wide range of activities to a city faced with a myriad of impediments to good health. The participants defined such primary target areas as provision of clean water and improved sanitation, control and protection of food services, environmental control, reforestation, control of prevalent risk factors and control of domestic animals. Targets were also set to increase urban services, develop municipal health promotion plans, and initiate projects related to mental health, citizen protection and health education.

An innovative programme to educate schoolchildren on urban problems and solutions has already been launched in La Paz. The objective of the programme is to facilitate student understanding of the urban development problems faced by their city. Children are encouraged to have a greater sensitivity for the challenges presented to them and their fellow community members by their environmental conditions. Project activities promote a critical but motivated attitude that will stimulate students to develop concrete solutions to the problems they face in their urban environment. These consciousness-raising activities parallel educational efforts that are already being carried out in the schools.

One of the main strategies the project uses to promote greater awareness is to transport the students by minibus throughout the city, concentrating particularly on the areas where students see first hand some of the city's major urban development problems. After the trips, students discuss these problems and propose solutions. Another strategy is to present students with an audio-visual expression of their urban reality through photographs, videos and models. Again, problems and potential solutions are debated. The children's discussions focus on issues such as proper waste disposal and the supply of clean water – crucial prerequisites for a community's good health. Food services are also discussed. Issues surrounding production, preservation, storage, transportation and sale of food are important to a city such as La Paz, where much food is prepared and sold on the street. Children also discuss ecologically sound and structurally safe housing facilities.

Yet another strategy used to educate young children is to bring them to specific park areas set aside for their recreation. During a full-day session the children participate in discussions about factors that damage their environment, such as air, water and land pollution. The children then try to develop preventive measures that could be taken to stop the destruction. Students in this and the other programmes are encouraged to do their own research to identify urban problems and solutions, as well as to inform and educate their families, friends and neighbours.

As evidenced by the activities described above, youth are another vital resource whose energy can be used to promote health in an urban context. Within schools and communities, youths have been successfully mobilized to promote the health of their neighbourhoods in many Third World cities. Youth groups have been organized, and many have applied themselves to the promotion of health within their cities. For example, the Bjarat Scouts and Guides in Delhi, India, adopted an action plan to improve the health conditions of their city, by carrying out construction and upgrading work as well as promoting sanitation. With help from UNICEF they helped set up demonstration sanitation units, and produced a sanitation promotion book which offers guidelines for individuals, and for groups. Several groups dug boreholes in poorer areas as part of their activities. Rangers and Rovers from all over India helped level roads, clear away rubbish, provide or improve drainage, and soak pits – and they went from house to house speaking to the residents about sanitation and other health matters (UNCHS 1988c).

Scouts in Mexico used money received from other Girl Guide and Girl Scout organizations to help a community which suffered considerable damage during the September 1985 earthquake. Many of the homes in the community of Delicias were either destroyed or so severely damaged as to be uninhabitable. The guides have undertaken plans to help rebuild the neighbourhood with larger communal areas, improved sanitary conditions and more light and space (UNCHS 1988c).

Another country where the Healthy Cities initiative has taken root with full force is Costa Rica. Throughout many neighbourhoods in many cities, communities are organizing to improve their health conditions. For example in the district of San Roque in the Barba Canton, a group of voluntary health promoters existed, composed of twenty community members, a doctor, a pharmacist, and a social worker. The group formed a team to clarify the concept of health in San Roque, and to identify the specific health problems their community faced. As a result of their discussions, the team chose environmental contamination as its priority challenge, defining it as 'a set of negative factors that exist in the San Roque environment that affect health'. Team members found abounding examples of this contamination resulting from practices such as burning garbage, abusing insecticides and inorganic fertilizers, and leaving animals unpenned. They also noted that garbage is not well collected, sewers are not maintained, coffee grounds are not disposed of, bathrooms are unsanitary, cars give off excess smoke, unpenned animals wander through the streets, and street vendors practise poor hygiene. In order to attack some of these problems, the group worked to develop programmes and strategies. Some of the projects underway include the installation of community garbage cans, publication of an educational bulletin, and a community drawing contest on relevant themes.

The activities in San Roque have also brought about other less visible but equally important improvements. An effective group, capable of generating knowledge and transmitting it to the community has been organized. This group, made up of many who do not traditionally participate in health activities, has already elaborated a more accurate concept of health in San Roque. It has awakened among many community members an interest in the participatory process and has created greater links and partnerships between institutions and the community. Through this process and these links, San Roque will continue to discover and use its community resources better to improve the city's health.

Several cities in the Caribbean have organized to confront the problem of death due to traffic accidents. In Jamaica, it was decided that the prevention of road traffic accidents and the resulting injuries and deaths demanded new ways of thinking. Traditionally, treatment, education, enforcement, legislation, infrastructural development and research programmes have operated in isolation of each other. It was felt that improved linkages of these efforts would provide significant assistance in improving the problem. An intersectoral steering committee called the 'National Safety Committee' was set up to manage the project, consisting of medical officers, insurance company representatives, the president of the National Safety Council, a research officer and others. The group then set out to implement a programme through a partnership of many sectors aimed at reducing the high number of traffic accidents by promoting road safety and educating selected groups on the subject. Both 14-year-old students from fourteen different high schools and representatives from identified health committees were trained to implement the educational aspect of the programme, and they prepared a traffic booklet for all schools involved in the programme.

In Rio de Janeiro, in the heart of one of its poorest neighbourhoods, the accomplishments of another organized group can already be seen. The community association called 'Asociación Rocinha' has united a community of roughly 80,000 persons and has initiated a wide spectrum of activities, ranging from establishing a system of garbage collection to organizing kindergartens. By dividing themselves into working committees for sanitation, health and education, the residents of the Rocinha neighbourhood have learned how to work together as well as how to work with the local bureaucracy to accomplish group goals. Jose Martins de Oliveira, head of the Sanitation Committee, said:

> We have learned how to negotiate with the bureaucracy. Now we go to the Municipal Secretary and say 'Give us the material we need, and we'll carry out the project'.
>
> (Murphy 1983)

In countries where government resources are sometimes insufficient to address the problems many urban residents face, this organization and community involvement is critical to accomplishing neighbourhood goals. The Rocinha Association has also solicited and received co-operation and support from religious, non-profit and international groups.

The groups' activities address many of the urban problems outlined earlier. In the area of education, teacher training programmes help to improve the quality of education the children receive, while a building renovation project works to improve the actual school-buildings. Kindergartens have also been established. An information system helps educate residents on health topics, while the sanitation committee works to improve the residents' environmental health conditions. One of these projects was to rebuild an open water and sewer system and install spillways for the waste of residents who live in higher areas of the neighbourhood. The work is done voluntarily by community members, many of whom are construction workers (Murphy 1983). The Rocinha policy is based upon community opinion and participation. Key policy elements include trust in the decision-making ability of the community, recruitment of local residents for part-time work, and a commitment to serve as co-ordinator between community groups and governmental bodies.

The 'Rocinha model' was so successful, it is now being used in other neighbourhoods of Rio de Janeiro. The community of Morro da Dona Marta, a poor neighbourhood in the hills near Rio, is another community which has begun to organize. This community has built a new 7,000 litre water storage tank with seven faucets and 45 metres of tubing, which now provides water to dozens of neighbourhood residents. Before this was built, residents had to walk far down the hill to water-canals, and carry the water back on foot. The system was installed by local residents who worked on weekends and holidays, using materials acquired from suppliers of local construction companies. The work was organized by the 'Bloco Carnavalesco Imperio de Botafogo', a samba song and dance group that normally devotes itself to helping the community prepare for Carnival festivities, but which is now becoming involved in a growing number of community activities (Murphy 1983).

Women's participation

In the developing world, urban poverty is becoming increasingly 'feminized'; this is highly visible in the slums and squatter settlements of developing countries, where women and children form the majority of residents. Women also contribute substantially to development. Therefore efforts that bring them into the mainstream of activities and decision-making are both necessary and effective (UNCHS 1988d).

The participation of women in project planning and implementation is a key element to the success of many efforts to improve urban health conditions in the developing world. The importance of involving women more actively in projects becomes more urgent when one considers that in the less developed world most of the recipients and providers of health care are women. Women not only gain from community health efforts, but also, as the principal influence on family health habits, they can greatly contribute to the better planning, functioning and utilization of health services and facilities. Furthermore, women make up at least 50 per cent of community populations and often comprise a larger part when their men migrate to seek work. Many urban households are headed by single women, giving them an even greater responsibility for, and involvement in, the health of their families. They and the organizations in which they participate make up a potentially valuable, but much under-utilized resource to accomplish the Healthy Cities objectives in the developing world.

The Baldia project in Karachi, Pakistan is an example of a successful attempt to improve sanitation in a slum area, which relied heavily on the initiative of women. Since the project was launched, 70 per cent of the households built soak-pit latrines. The initiative for latrines often comes from women. It is women who suffer most inconvenience when there are no toilet facilities in the home. It is also women who have to take care of the needs of their children and any ageing household relative. Almost half of the work of constructing latrines was undertaken by women; all the health committees formed have women representatives among their most active members (Yansheng and Elmendorf 1984).

In Honduras, at the suggestion of a women's legal society in Tegucigalpa, barrio women enlarged their group to a community-wide action committee headed by women. They made a formal request to the city authorities to get four standpipes installed in their hillside slum. They put two standpipes near the top of the hill and two near the bottom, protected by little wooden shacks. One of each pair is open five hours a day in the morning, and the other five hours in the afternoon. A community woman, usually from a female-headed household, is hired by the committee on a rota basis to be in charge of the standpipes, to collect set fees for water and to keep the water sites clean (Yansheng and Elmendorf 1984).

The Popular Unity Co-operative in El Puyo, the main town in Ecuador's Amazon region, undertook a low-income housing project involving three phases. Women were not admitted to the first or the second phases, which required manual lifting of 40 to 50 kilograms per person. However, in the third phase 70 per cent of the membership in the co-operative were women, and the programme remained under their control (UNCHS 1988b). From the start of the programme, women were especially active in not only organizational tasks but also the heaviest work such as site preparation and the production of foundation components, as well as actual building. Of all the activities in which the women were involved the most impressive was the production of foundation components. It was not a traditional area of work for them; it involved steel-bending and moulding the components. Later they made blocks for the fire-resistant walls. This then became the starting-point for a small block production firm of which the women were in charge.

Until December 1985, eight women worked in shifts to turn out blocks. The way in which the group was organized was in complete contrast to that of the men. While the latter's building components, workshop, construction and assembly teams were of the traditional hierarchical type (manager, supervisor, foremen, etc.) the women established a horizontal form of organization. Responsibilities were shared equally, both in the administration of the workshop and actual physical activity. Income grew and the small firm expanded (UNCHS 1988b).

The construction of their own homes, a day nursery and a social centre showed the women the purpose of their own contribution to these activities. This led to the start of group training by the women themselves. From the training and their practical experience, members saw that they were involved in a productive activity which could possibly provide a source of income and stable employment.

Conclusions

The future growth of Healthy Communities in the Third World depends on the expansion of activities similar to those outlined above. The variety and degree of health problems faced by urban residents of the Third World seem at first glance to pose a challenge of herculean dimensions. Populations are exploding, environments are becoming ever more unhealthy, and economic resources with which to combat these problems are stagnating and in some cases even shrinking. Yet within this difficult context, many communities have successfully worked to define their priorities and improve the environment in which they live. Residents need to be more aware of the highest priority health problems and conditions in their community. However, even in some cases when they are aware what is most needed is a catalyst to facilitate the formation of partnerships and coalitions that will enable communities to solve their own problems.

The communities of Favela do Gato in Brazil, El Puyo in Ecuador, San

Roque in Costa Rica, and many others all provide models for successful community organization and health action within the developing world. These communities, recognizing the collective nature of their health problems, worked collectively to overcome them. Recognizing the scarcity of resources available through traditional channels (namely government funding), they sought and found their own resources. These resources often appeared in the form of labour, skills and enthusiasm from within the communities themselves. Participants included women, youths, existing community organizations and newly formed groups. The time has come for the politicians, governments and formal institutions to recognize their responsibilities in supporting efforts such as these, and wherever possible, to serve as the needed catalyst to initiate Healthy Cities activities that will become self-sustaining and mutually reinforcing.

References and further reading

Adegbola, O. (1987) 'The Impact of Urbanization and Industrialization on Health Conditions: The Case of Nigeria', *World Health Statistics Quarterly* 40: 74.
Baldi, P. (1988) 'Increasing Global Interdependence: Population, Environment, and Food', Paper presented to Global Development Conference, 16 April.
Bruntland, G. (1990) 'In Tune with Nature', *World Health* January–February: 4.
Canedo, M., Elisa, M. and Bienenstein, R. (1985) *Community Participation in Brazil: Case Study – Favela Do Gato*, Occasional Papers in Planning no. 9, Department of Country Planning, The Queen's University of Belfast.
Cornia, G.A., Jolly, R. and Stewart, F. (eds) (1989) *Adjustment with a Human Face, Volume 1: Protecting the Vulnerable and Promoting Growth*, Oxford: Clarendon Press.
Duhl, L. (1990) 'Health and the City', *World Health* January–February: 10–12.
Hardoy, J.E. and Satterthwaite, D.E. (1987) 'Las Ciudades del Tercer Mundo y el Medio Ambiente de Pobreza', *Foro Mundial de la Salud* 8: 87–96.
Jensen, L. (1989) 'A Thai Alternative to Slum Clearance', *World Development* January: 14–17.
Kreisel, W. (1990) 'Environmental Health in 1990s', *World Health* January–February: 5.
Lopez, A.D. (1987) 'The Impact of Demographic Trends on Health: Introduction', *World Health Statistics Quarterly* 40: 2.
Murphy, T. (1983) 'Son los pobres los que hacen que sea lo que es', *Noticias del Unicef* 115: 14–16.
Musgrove, P. (1987) 'The Economic Crisis and its Impact on Health and Health Care in Latin America and the Caribbean', *International Journal of Health Services* 17(3): 411.
Oakley, P. (1989) *Community Involvement in Health Development: An Examination of the Critical Issues*, Geneva: World Health Organization.
Organizacion Panamericana de la Salud (1988) *Orientaciones para el Desarrollo de Proyectos Investigacion-Accion Participativa*, Serie Desarrollo de Servicios de Salud Numero 66, Organizacion Panamericana de la Salud.
Paganini, J.M. (1989) 'La Salud en las Grandes Ciudades y los Sistemas Locales de Salud', *Boletin de la Oficina Panamerica de la Salud*, 107(1): 65–73.
Pan American Health Organization (1988) *Social Participation in Local Health*

Systems, Health Services Development Series no. 35, Washington: Pan American Health Organization.

Pan American Health Organization (forthcoming) *Health Conditions in the Americas, 1985–1988*, Scientific Publications, Washington: Pan American Health Organization.

Project Hope (1989) 'Child Survival in Honduras', *HOPE* 27(1): 1–5.

Rice, M. (1990) *Social Participation and SILOS*, Washington: Pan American Health Organization.

Tolley, G.S. and Vinod, T. (eds) (1987) *The Economics of Urbanization and Urban Policies in Developing Countries*, Washington: World Bank.

UNCHS (Habitat) (1988a) 'Towards a Healthy Habitat', *UNCHS (Habitat) Shelter Bulletin* 1(2): 4–5.

UNCHS (Habitat) (1988b) 'Ecuador – A Co-operative Project Involving women', *UNCHS (Habitat) Shelter Bulletin* 1(2): 8.

UNCHS (Habitat) (1988c) 'Scouts/Guides Active in Shelter Activities', *UNCHS (Habitat) Shelter Bulletin* 1(2): 11.

UNCHS (Habitat) (1988d) 'Women and the Global Human Environment', *Habitat News* 10(2): 4.

United Nations (1986) *World Population Trends and Policies: 1987 Monitoring Report*, New York: United Nations.

Welna, D. (1988) 'Housing Solutions for Buenos Aires' Invisible Poor', *Grassroots Development* 12(1): 2–7.

Yansheng, Ma and Elmendorf, M. (1984) 'Insights from Field Practice: How Women Have Been and Could Be Involved in Water and Sanitation at the Community Level', *Background Paper V*, Inter-Agency Task Force on Women and Water of the Steering Committee for Cooperative Action of the IDWSSD: 1–17.

III

European case studies

10

Liverpool

Geoffrey Green

For a century Liverpool was one of the world's great ports and one of its largest slums. The city's prosperous and confident merchants were the first in the world to appoint a City Medical Officer of Health to control death and disease in the population of this insanitary environment, the first to appoint a City Engineer to build the water and sewage system. The city helped create the first Public Health movement which transformed city landscapes in a series of improvements to water, work-places, air and housing.

Liverpool has also helped to create the new Public Health and the idea of a Healthy City. In this new phase of interest in Public Health, the city is one of the poorest in Western Europe, on the edge of economic viability, on the verge of municipal bankruptcy. The new Public Health comes from a radically different combination of economic, social and environmental forces, grouped around decline rather than prosperity. Enumerating this relative deprivation was perhaps the first of three important influences on the Healthy City idea. In the early 1980s it became possible to construct a new epidemiology of poverty and death. Many UK cities described the geography in health inequality within their boundaries with death-rates in the poorest districts no better than the UK average forty years earlier when the National Health Service was founded (in 1948). We could also compare cities, and Liverpool compared badly, vying for lung cancer capital of the world. This had a big impact on Labour politicians especially. Stoutly defending the principle of equal access to what had become a National Sickness Service, they had neglected equality of health outcome. Now was the opportunity to put equity in health back on the agenda.

Second, by overcoming enormous political problems, Liverpool achieved an early partnership between key city agencies for the Healthy Cities initiative. In the 1980s city administrations of great northern cities in the UK were in political conflict with a Conservative central government over resources, local democracy and the value of public services. In so far as local health services are run by central government, there was conflict there also. It was especially acute in Liverpool which had a left-wing Militant council allied to strong public sector trade unions. The Healthy City initiative transcended the conflict by emphasizing health outcomes broadly defined, rather than health services defined by jobs and resources. It took further effort primarily by officers in the key agencies to turn potential common ground into creative partnership. But it was achieved by 1987 and has been sustained without conflict as perhaps the only regular meeting of the key city authorities.

Third, from Liverpool University's Department of Public Health, John Ashton and others led the UK in developing an international vision of a Healthy City as a focus for the earlier concept of Health for All. Since 1986 the idea has gained great momentum in many towns and cities across the UK. It cuts across party politics and cross-cuts Green politics. A Conservative government at least tolerates it. The Opposition Labour Party now aligned with progressive European social movements and institutions welcomes it, both in content (cf. policy documents) and because it reinforces British social democracy as part of mainstream Europe. Similarly Labour-controlled municipalities, beleaguered and devalued by central government, welcome it both as an inspiration and as endorsement for their environmental and social policies. It is yet to be tested in the operational theatre of conflicting programmes and plans. But it is at least an idea whose time has come.

The project organization

To turn an idea into a project, Liverpool applied to WHO for designation as a participating city in their European initiative. Liverpool was chosen in Lisbon in 1986, undemocratically alongside a slice of London called Camden or Bloomsbury. Other cities and towns, which expressed an interest, have yet to work out how it was done, and were initially resentful that the process would create a two-tier system in the UK. In the event, many moved ahead rapidly without formal WHO support. Liverpool faltered. An impressive intersectoral committee had been formed in 1987 from ten partner agencies. It was supported by a highly proficient technical committee of officers and professionals. They secured finance for a series of model projects and for an office and executive team of three, bigger and potentially more effective than any other UK city. And the March 1988 international conference sustained the idea. Then there was a long hiatus: staff appointments were delayed, the technical committee suspended work and the intersectoral committee did not meet.

It was another year before the project was fully operational, then a further year getting organized for an ambitious programme. It was not easy; nor, according to WHO's mid-term assessment (June 1990), very successful. At a mundane level the usual problems of setting up an office were compounded by the nightmare bureaucracy of Liverpool City Council which had agreed to host the project. A great amount of energy was consumed, turning an attic slum into offices, skirting the council's financial crises with a health authority grant to secure running costs and a communications budget, overcoming restrictive employment and Information Technology (IT) practices to get an efficient secretariat. There was frustration also from the owners of the project. The number of partner agencies expanded to fourteen and their senior representatives remain more or less committed, but the technical committee of officers, sector facilitators, uncertain of their role, dissolved in mid-1990. We reorganized so that their executive and representational functions are now clearly separated. Community and voluntary sector representatives are asked to contribute instead to topic forums (following Glasgow's example) and these, in turn, will elect representatives to the intersectoral committee. The project team is now more clearly the executive, strengthened by key officers from the partner agencies who can give time as well as commitment. After a year or two of frustration, the stage is now set and the resources lined up for a grand production.

Strategy for change

'*Think globally; act locally*' really does determine our overall strategy. The Liverpool Declaration which committed Liverpool's key partner authorities at the May 1988 Conference is based on international principles of 'Health for All' see Appendix at the end of this chapter. The Liverpool intersectoral committee itself is recognition of WHO's 1978 Alma Ata Declaration that health requires action across all sectors. Our city health planning process is structured around the thirty-eight European Regional Targets for Health for All. Our view of Liverpool's people as a resource for health (and not merely the passive recipients of health services) borrows from WHO's 1986 Ottawa Charter for Health Promotion. And finally the European Healthy Cities initiative transcends local conflict over the National Health Service with a broad concept of health as a focus for partnership and civic pride. In the best-laid plans, health is integral to the regeneration of one of Western Europe's poorest and unhealthiest cities.

Such declarations of intent inspire and motivate. But down-to-earth, many of these ideals cannot be attained in the foreseeable future. So our realistic objective is a measurable improvement by the year 2000 in Liverpool's health relative to the UK and Europe, and an even greater improvement in Liverpool's poorer districts. This will not be achieved by project staff alone. Ultimately it is the responsibility of Liverpool's citizens and the key authorities who are partners to the intersectoral committee. Only they can deliver the plans and programmes, find the resources and run the service. If the foundations are in place in the early 1990s, improvements in lifestyle, environment and care will surely follow in the mid-1990s, leading to a measurable improvement in Liverpool's health by 2000. The modest aim of the project is to begin this process. Our role is to lead, enable, facilitate, support, communicate, demonstrate, influence and eventually create the preconditions for others to deliver.

Programme

How does this work in practice? With, we hope, a magical combination which gives equal weight to both health outcomes and the process of change. On the one hand, we have sought to develop city-wide plans and targets within a Health for All framework; on the other, we encourage 1,000 flowers to bloom, taking opportunities where we can, aligning with the current agendas and priorities, feelings and fears of partners and communities.

Once the project was underway in 1989, the intersectoral committee moved quickly to adopt a programme of work guided by *Targets for Health for All* (WHO 1985). We borrowed both the European model of change and the timetable to the year 2000, while resisting imprisonment by the specific targets themselves. *Targets for Health for All* addresses nation-states. We adapt it to a city. Our focus is a City Health Plan, negotiated and agreed by partner agencies and the public of Liverpool by 1991. It will be built from components, the six target blocks – health, lifestyles, the environment, appropriate care, research, development – providing the essential structure. The process of arriving is as important as the plan itself. We specified a seven-stage process originally, starting with a draft for each of the thirty-eight target areas, giving a picture of Liverpool, the strategies for change and projections towards the year 2000. Then we plan to consult, refine, negotiate and refine again.

Of course it hasn't run as smoothly or evenly as envisaged. At the end of 1990 some target areas were neglected. But others had attracted great debate and widened the circle of participants to 300. Sometimes we proceeded by workshops, then write-ups – the Water Workshops under the chandeliers of the old Town Hall, multisectoral policies for the environment in the University's Department of Civic Design. Mostly it was done by working groups of professionals, convened by an active member of the partnership – appropriate care by a consultant in public health (Targets 26–32), lifestyles by a health promotion officer (Targets 13–17). Suicide prevention (Target 12) was completed brilliantly in three weeks by a team of students from the School of Tropical Medicine. But however the information was gained, the next step is publication of accessible yet authoritative pamphlets, leaflets, brochures and a series of workshops, seminars and conferences. Initially they will revolve around specific target areas, components of the plan, but the whole, the vision of Liverpool as a Healthy City, is never far away.

A series of model projects complement the broader planning process. The first three were on the drawing board in 1988. They are designed with a research element so that we can draw on their experience for the city as a whole. Equally they are action programmes in their own right with short term successes and failures. The YUK poisoning campaign was the first under the Healthy Cities banner. Launched in 1989, managed by the City's Environmental Health Department, with symbols adapted from Philadelphia, it aims to reduce accidental poisoning in children. Second is the Health and Fitness Point accessible to office and shop workers through a city centre shop-front. Users are tested for fitness and health then given prescriptions for sport and recreation which will improve their condition. With occupational sickness in Liverpool much higher than the national average the service benefits employee and employer alike. Initially funded by the City Council's Urban Programme and managed by their Sport and Recreation Division, it should, in time, attract private sector funding especially if research demonstrates that it really does improve lifestyles (Targets 15–17).

The third and biggest project so far is the Croxteth Health Action Area (the first in the UK) based on two poor council estates in an outer suburb of the city. The area was chosen because a residents' report in the early 1980s said poor housing was the biggest cause of ill health. Our initial research confirmed that substantial housing improvements since then have improved residents' health. The aim of the project is to involve residents actively in the other aspects of the physical and social environment. A neighbourhood health team moved into the area early in 1990 to provide a nucleus of energy and support. They will try to reform the delivery of formal health and social services to the area. Their primary aim, however, is to activate the skills and resources of the community itself. In most surveys, family, neighbours and friends account for 90 per cent of the balance of community care. Our presumption is that illness prevention and health promotion is also largely in the hands of the community itself. As the neighbourhood team themselves put it

> The project can, and intends to, achieve the strengthening, development and extension of existing social, economic and environmental structures within the Community. These are associated with the intermediate WHO Targets to be achieved by the mid-1990s – improvements in Lifestyle (Targets 13–17), in the Environment (Targets 18–25), in Appropriate Care (Targets 26–31). These provide the foundations enabling people to make and support their personal choices and preferences. People do not choose to impair or damage their health. Their options are limited. What is seen as unwise or inappropriate lifestyle is, in reality, a strategy for survival, adapting and coping in an environment which is hostile and unsupportive of good health practices and regimes. Creating a supportive environment is the primary aim of the health action area project.

Appendix

WORLD HEALTH ORGANISATION
HEALTHY CITIES PROJECT

THE LIVERPOOL DECLARATION
ON THE RIGHT TO HEALTH

Equity in Health

Community Participation

Partnerships for Health

Health Promotion

Primary Health Care

Research for Health

International co-operation

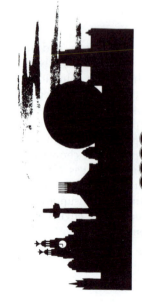

HEALTH FOR ALL

The Liverpool Declaration was produced by the Healthy Cities Inter-Sectoral
Committee, for ratification at the UK HEALTHY CITIES CONFERENCE held in
Liverpool on 28-30 March, 1988

THE LIVERPOOL DECLARATION

"At least I know this, that if a person is overworked in any degree they
cannot enjoy the sort of health I am speaking of: nor if they are continually
chained to one dull round of mechanical work, with no hope at the other
end of it; nor if they live in continual sordid anxiety for their livelihood; nor if
they are ill housed; nor if they are deprived of all enjoyment of the natural
beauty of the world; nor if they have no amusement to quicken the flow of
their spirits from time to time; all these things, which touch more or less
directly on their bodily condition, are born of the claim I make to live in
good health".

William Morris, 1884

BACKGROUND

The UK Healthy Cities Conference was planned by the agencies whose
collaboration forms the basis of Liverpool's involvement in the World
Health Organisations (WHO) Healthy Cities Project. Its purpose was to bring
together people from towns and cities in the UK to share ideas and
experiences in setting an agenda for **the new public health** in urban
situations. Two major aspects of this aim are the development of
collaborative **healthy city plans** and the promotion of a **healthy cities
network** of UK towns and cities committed to achieving health for all their
citizens. This Declaration represents a third aspect: Liverpool's agenda for
the new public health.

PRINCIPLES OF HEALTH FOR ALL

In seeking to achieve health for all citizens of the United Kingdom, we
acknowledge and confirm these fundamental principles, expressed in
the WHO "Global Strategy for Health for All by the Year 2000" (1981) and
the WHO European Region "Targets For Health For All" (1985).

THE RIGHT TO HEALTH
Health is a fundamental human right and a worldwide social goal.

EQUITY IN HEALTH
The existing gross inequality in the health status of people is of common
concern to all countries and must be drastically reduced.

COMMUNITY PARTICIPATION
People have the right and the duty to participate individually and
collectively in the planning and implementation of their health care.

INTERSECTORAL COLLABORATION
Governments have a responsibility for the health of their people which
can be fulfilled only by the provision of adequate health and other social
measures. The political commitment of the State as a whole, and not
merely the ministry of health, is essential to the attainment of health for all.

HEALTH PROMOTION
The starting point in changing lifestyles depends to a
considerable extent health depends on the political, social, cultural,
economic and physical environment. The first aim is therefore to provide
opportunities and develop capacities for adopting healthy lifestyles.

PRIMARY HEALTH CARE

Primary health care forms an integral part both of the country's health system, of which it is the central function and main focus, and of the overall social and economic development of the community.

INTERNATIONAL COOPERATION

Where health is concerned no country is self-sufficient; international solidarity is required to ensure the development and implementation of health strategies and to overcome obstacles.

In addition to describing the principles of Health For All, the WHO Global Strategy reminds us that "In conformity with the recognition by the United Nations General Assembly of health as an integral part of development, the human energy generated by improved health should be channelled into sustaining economic and social development, and economic and social development should be harnessed to improve the health of people".

TURNING PRINCIPLES INTO ACTIONS

THE RIGHT TO HEALTH

In recognising every citizen's **right** to good health, we accept the **responsibility** carried by all agencies, throughout our society, to take account of the public health costs of all their activities.

Practically all of the activities of agencies in our society can affect the public health. Such agencies include central and local government, health and education authorities, the non-statutory sector, employers, landlords, academic bodies: the churches, communicators; everyone taking part in the production and consumption of our goods and services, our values and attitudes. If health for all is to be achieved we must complement the economic audit which accounts for the financial costs of these activities with a social audit which assesses their health and other human costs. Without this social accounting for the health costs of public and private decisions, the right to health is an empty goal.

EQUITY IN HEALTH — THE REDUCTION OF INEQUALITY

We reject all forms of discrimination that reduce people's chances of good health, and accept the challenge of substantially reducing current health inequalities.

There are many aspects of people's lives which contribute to the substantial and increasing health inequalities in the United Kingdom. These include, amongst others, their sex, their social class, their skin colour,

their area of residence, their physical abilities and their sexual orientation. In asserting people's rights to equity in health, we assert also their rights to fairness of treatment in all of these areas. These rights include their access to:

- adequate income, in or out of paid employment
- safe, warm, sound, affordable housing
- healthy, cheap, accessible food
- worthwhile, safe, properly rewarded work
- cheap, ecologically sound public and private transport
- freedom from sexual or racial harassment
- equal respect regardless of personal circumstances
- safe, planned, health enhancing environments
- leisure facilities and social support networks
- comprehensive, properly resourced public services

In actively promoting these rights we will work towards major reductions in the current inequalities in health.

COMMUNITY PARTICIPATION

We acknowledge the necessity for meaningful public participation in all processes and activities that affect people's health.

Health for all cannot be achieved without participation by all. A crucial element in becoming healthy is taking control over one's life. This has to involve empowering people by offering them a voice in the decisions that affect their health. Among other things, it implies opening up the membership of all bodies, at all levels, which take such decisions within the public sector; legislation may be necessary to achieve full participation. Decentralising management structures can be an important prelude to inviting participation. Policy decisions should also be informed by surveys of public attitudes and priorities. Empowering individuals to take part in activities affecting their health involves choosing policies and allocating resources that make the healthiest choices the easiest choices; once we have achieved this, any necessary educational processes are straightforward. In seeking participation, however, we also acknowledge the freedom of people to make choices and hold views on health with which we disagree.

INTERSECTORAL COLLABORATION — PARTNERSHIPS FOR HEALTH

We will work with all agencies and groups whose activities are relevant to the promotion of the public health.

Most of the major influences on health lie beyond the scope of health services. Despite this fact, there has been little real shared development between agencies at central or local levels of plans and strategies for promoting public health. We acknowledge the need for genuine joint planning for health for all; this must start from a consideration of the health needs of the people and 'work backwards' to the institutional means of meeting them. Such a joint approach to public health is required both between government departments and between local agencies and groups.

HEALTH PROMOTION

We acknowledge our collective responsibility to promote and create healthy physical and social environments, and to facilitate peoples' choices of healthy lives.

Health promotion is a constant theme in public policy, since both are concerned with improving the quality of peoples' lives. We must be active in promoting awareness of this fact, and in working to make healthy the environments in which people live, work and enjoy leisure. People must also be given the resources and the information to make healthy choices. This involves a sensitive understanding of the responses of different social groups: traditional health promotion has often required increased social inequalities in health.

PRIMARY HEALTH CARE

Primary health care must become the central function and main focus of our national health service.

Primary health care is the promotion of health and the provision of health care within communities. It is based on **active partnerships** between primary health care workers and the people, and on **teamwork** between primary health care workers. It should provide all but the most specialised elements of health care, and hence should be the main focus of health systems. In order to achieve these aspirations, embodied in the Declaration of Alma-Ata, we will strive towards:

* the direction of new resources toward primary health care
* the demystification of primary health care through patient participation groups, self-help groups, libraries, courses and other community resources in health centres
* the promotion of teamwork between all primary health care workers
* the provision of services sensitive to peoples' needs such as well person clinics, nurse practitioners and community health workers
* localising the organisation and planning of primary health care to the neighbourhood level

INTERNATIONAL COOPERATION

As health promoters in a rich nation, we acknowledge our shared responsibility for the health of the world.

We wish to play a full role in Healthy Cities and other WHO networks which contribute to the health of all the world's peoples. In addition to material aid, we can fulfil this role:

* by actively opposing the export of unhealthy products
* by resisting the export by UK interests of practices harmful to the health of people in other countries, such as unsafe working conditions, inappropriate promotion of drugs or baby foods
* by protecting and providing for the health of migrant workers, refugees and victims of torture who come to the UK

RESEARCH

We will encourage in all relevant ways the research necessary to achieve health for all.

We shall not achieve our goals without considerable developments in researching the public health. Much work is required if we are fully to understand the nature of the many inequalities in health. The development of social audit, accounting and investment poses a major challenge. Little is understood of the mechanisms of community participation in health. Joint approaches to public health planning and to healthy public policy require evaluation. If we are to move towards primary **health care** (and away from primary **medical care**), we must first demonstrate its greater effectiveness.

As well as new research **agendas**, health for all requires new styles of research, such as participatory methods which involve the affected communities in the design, implementation and action stages of research into their health; and research instruments which are sensitive to peoples' own health perspectives. Monitoring and surveillance of the public health will require new measures and indicators. All of the above will together constitute the development of **a new social epidemiology** which will refocus away from the diseases of groups of individuals and towards the health of populations. And of course, this development will not occur without the allocation of the necessary resources.

We seek the support of all people of the United Kingdom for this Declaration. We are sure that with that support, we can move confidently towards health for all.

References

WHO (World Health Organization) (1978) *Alma Ata 1977. Primary Health Care*, Geneva: WHO/UNICEF.
WHO Europe (1985) *Targets in Support of the European Strategy for Health for All*, Geneva: WHO.
WHO, Health and Welfare Canada, Canadian Public Health Association (1986) *Ottawa Charter for Health Promotion*, Copenhagan: WHO.

11

Sheffield

Gavin Thoms

'Healthy Sheffield 2000' is the city's unifying initiative for the interpretation of Health for All, and it has been backed by the major organizations in Sheffield since 1986. It has three major benefits: its organizational structure links many agencies in the city; it provides the framework for a number of operational health promotion projects; and it focuses the development of a strategy for Health for All (HFA) that makes sense at the level of the whole city.

Although the initiative has increased in complexity since its launch, three key aims in the original vision remain unchanged:

1 To establish collaboration and coalitions, involving a wide range of individuals and organizations.
2 To apply the principles of Health for All.
3 To ensure that a health strategy for Sheffield is locally developed and locally owned.

Very early into the Project it became clear that satisfying this third aim would involve a major reworking of the HFA strategy for Europe.

This chapter first explains a little of the context in Sheffield in 1986. It goes on to describe:

1 How the initiative then grew.
2 Some of the early choices that shaped the project.
3 Why there has been a close look at the approach to our strategy, leading to a new shape for the local strategy for HFA.
4 Some of the operational programmes that have been developed within the Healthy Sheffield 2000 (HS2000) organization.
5 Something of the nature of the work involved in the initiative in 1989 and 1990.

Sheffield: the context in 1986

Sheffield is a large industrial city, with a population of around 530,000. The traditional industry is steel, and high-quality steel is still manufactured although on a greatly reduced scale in comparison with the first half of the century.

There is substantial male unemployment (up to 25 per cent in certain areas). In recent years major efforts backed by the City Council, Sheffield Development Corporation and local commerce have met with apparent success in attracting industries into the city, particularly into the East End area that was formerly the site of large-scale steelworks.

Sheffield has a history and local consciousness of preventive initiatives, including clean air developments in the 1960s and a major city-wide effort in the prevention of cot deaths. There is also a strong track record of planning and collaboration between the Health and Local Authorities, over a wide range of issues. In 1986 there was already a well-developed joint planning structure, the Joint Consultative Committee.

In terms of joint working in health promotion, Sheffield's strengths are as follows:

1 It is one of the biggest health districts in England in population terms although compact geographically.
2 It is relatively circumscribed. The Pennine hills are the boundary to the west and although there is travel to work (and flows of patients in) from the neighbouring towns of Barnsley and Rotherham to the north-east and Chesterfield to the south, this is on a small scale. Each town has its own transport system and the local media, apart from regional television, are Sheffield dominated.
3 The health authority and local authority have identical boundaries. This conveys an enormous advantage compared with those cities in which a number of small health authorities are required to share the responsibility of provision of health care, and need to relate to a single large local authority.

In 1985 the City Council commissioned Colin Thunhurst's report *Poverty and Health in the City of Sheffield*. The following year Sheffield Health Authority (1986) produced its *Health Care and Disease: A Profile of Sheffield*. These studies on the association between indicators of deprivation and of health experience followed the emergence of the Black Report (1980), *Inequalities in Health*, and led to substantial debate between the health and local authorities about the response that should be made. It appeared that there were 1,100 preventable deaths per year in the city, implying that even larger numbers were suffering from preventable illness. The pattern of ill health fitted closely with areas of deprivation. Those living in the well-off electoral wards of the city had a seven-year life expectation advantage over their neighbours in the deprived wards.

First steps towards a coalition

In 1986 discussion within the Joint Consultative Committee prompted by the Thunhurst Report (1985) had led to an acceptance of the existence of major inequities in preventable illness. The health authority identified health promotion as a major development area for its Public Health (then Community Medicine) Department. Also there was a growing acceptance by the health authority of the concept that the majority of opportunities for prevention lie outside the traditional activities of the Health Service. It became clear that there were unexploited opportunities for prevention that would arise from collaboration with other organizations, principally, but not exclusively, the local authority.

The Thunhurst Report had also created a climate of increased relevance and personal involvement in health promotion for city councillors and council officers. The Council's Environmental Health Department created a Health Promotion Research Unit, from a former education section, in recognition of the need for a new approach to public health.

So, at an organizational level, there was the beginning of a willingness to develop health promotion policy and programmes jointly. It became clear that this willingness also existed at an individual level: in several of the key departments of the Local and Health Authorities there were individuals of director or assistant director status who had the vision, capability and leeway within their own work programmes to take on the initiative. In July 1986 an intersectoral planning team (then known as the 'Sheffield 2000 Planning Team') was constituted as a joint team of officers reporting to the Sheffield Joint Consultative Committee. The organizations represented on the team are shown in Table 11.1.

The initial meetings of the Planning Team were concerned with trying to ascertain the existing and potential roles and responsibilities in health promotion of the various departments involved. A very early decision lay between taking stock of all existing initiatives and activities related to health promotion, and the alternative of setting out in a new direction. And, if the Planning Team were to take the latter course should this involve operational health promotion programmes (for example on topics such as health and nutrition, smoking, heart disease prevention, women's health, and AIDS education)? Or would energy be better invested in arriving at a joint health strategy for the city, serving to unite organizations in their vision for health, and therefore changing the way they plan? This decision concerning the initial investment of the time and energy of a small number of health promotion workers was a turnkey issue for the shape of the Healthy Sheffield Initiative.

The team agreed to work first at the level of strategy, and later to foster operational programmes on specific health promotion topics, against the background of an agreed strategy. The reason was a concern that programmes based solely on health promotion topics might be vulnerable to changes in policy or funding availability in parent organizations. We needed the safeguard of a unifying grand plan, of which such programmes would form an essential part.

At this time, the WHO European targets for Health for All were being increasingly promoted and the European office of WHO launched the Healthy Cities Initiative. The Sheffield 2000 Health Planning Team saw that the European targets for HFA provided a major opportunity for launching a local strategy. In mid-1987, the now renamed Healthy Sheffield 2000 Planning Team launched a set of local targets for Health for All. These Sheffield targets were fronted by a brochure which explained both the level of health inequities in the city, and also some of the links between the causes and effects of ill health. It summarized the proposed WHO approach including the principles of Health for All, demystifying the concept of targets for health. Thirty thousand of these brochures were distributed across the city using a variety of distribution routes, the launch securing local, regional and national news coverage with penetration into professional journals.

Table 11.1 Organizations and departments represented on the Healthy Sheffield 2000 Planning Team

1986	*1988*	*1990*

THE HEALTH SERVICE:
Health Authority HQ
Family Practitioner
  Committee
	(also)
	Community Services Unit
	  Management
	Health Education
		(also)
		Hospital Unit
		  Management

LOCAL AUTHORITY: Central Policy Unit	(also) Housing, Education	(also intended) Department of Economic Development

Health and Consumer
  Services (Environmental
  Health)
	Social Services,
	Publicity, and Recreation	

VOLUNTARY:
Council for Voluntary
  Services
	(also)
	Council for Racial
	  Equality
	Community Health
	  Council	

		ACADEMIC: City Polytechnic Business School
		(also intended) University
		COMMERCE & INDUSTRY:
		(intended) World Student Games Chamber of Commerce Sheffield Partnerships

A second major strand of work in the early days of the initiative was the identification of resources:

1 To fund the necessary research, publicity, programme design and evaluation.
2 To set up a core worker, or team of workers, who could co-ordinate the initiative.
3 To support the specific operational health promotion programmes.

Some success with an application for public funding (joint finance) in 1987 provided core funding of £16,000 in 1988 and enabled a full-time co-ordinator to be established, which in turn enabled a phase of rapid acceleration to occur.

The following three sections of this chapter highlight the activities that have taken place since. They deal with: the local strategy development; the operational health promotion programmes; and the nature of the work for those at the centre of the initiative.

The Sheffield Health for All strategy

The 1987 proposed Sheffield targets were local refinements of the European targets. When possible numerical precision was added, although it has to be said that the numerical value attached to a target was often a best guess based upon a consensus of local experts. Local relevance was added by portraying the canvas on which changes would occur as being at city level. This was intended to encourage debate amongst local residents and their elected representatives for example on the subject of inequities in health chances and life expectation.

We also intended to ensure that debate occurred on the potential for health promotion and of a preventive approach to illness, across many organizations and groupings in the city. In the process we hoped to learn where and why there might be hostility and where there were allies.

Feedback was gained on a large scale. We started building up a picture of the relevance of a city-wide approach to health promotion for particular groups and organizations. And we began to learn about the changes that would have to be made to this first Sheffield attempt at a strategic approach to Health for All if we were to secure maximum support and involvement from Sheffield's professionals, organizations and individuals.

Indeed the scale of reactions made it quite impossible for the officers involved to deal with all of them and it is probable that a number of potentially important learning opportunities and coalitions that could have occurred in the wake of the launch, were lost through shortage of human resources.

The major finding from the dialogue was that there were, in the target approach, some flaws which would require substantial developmental work to remedy. In summary our respondents said:

1 To arrive at a local strategy which mainly emphasized targets was not particularly motivating for most respondents. Another way of portraying the potential for change, and the relevance for a wide range of organizations and individuals, would have to be achieved.
2 Some of the targets which make sense at European or country level do not reflect the main concerns at city level.
3 Those with expertise in child health and mental health felt that the thirty-eight European targets underrepresented these issues.
4 The targets found to be most easy to engage with, tend to be disease-based, leading to a bias against the apparent relevance of social issues, and perpetuating a mechanistic model of ill health.
5 There is inadequate attention given to the very major issue of the material resources necessary for acceptable levels of health, in contrast to the findings of the Sheffield reports that link deprivation and ill health.
6 If targets were to be used as the main content of a new city strategy for health, very much more development work would be required to demonstrate how targets should be achieved and by whom. The need to develop indicators demonstrating progress towards or away from health targets at city level was recognized.
7 Many came to see the targets as the main issue and purpose, losing all sight of the principles of Health for All. The team then embarked on a period of work in an attempt to improve the robustness of the arguments for and relevance of the thirty-eight adapted European targets.

Much of this approach was motivated by a timetable set by the parent organizations for bringing out a 'final' strategy.

However, it became clear that there were enormous difficulties in this task; by December 1988 we concluded that a completely different approach to a local strategy would be required. To be effective, the new strategy would have to deal adequately with the reactions that had been received to the initial draft strategy including those concerns listed above. And it would have to involve Sheffield organizations and people in its development and crafting.

So a new approach was developed in outline, and endorsed by the Healthy Sheffield 2000 (HS2000) Planning Team in June 1989. Although targets are still a feature, the intention since then has been to produce a strategic framework for public health which provides a practical planning tool for all city organizations that are concerned to optimize the health impact of their policies and activities. Objectives within the strategy will be developed participatively by the interested agencies. The strategy is being designed to be dynamic and capable of progressive refinement. Figure 11.1 shows the probable content of a Public Health Strategy Discussion Document for Sheffield.

HEALTH GOALS

- Women
- Men
- Children
- Older adults
- Young people
- Ethnic minorities
- People with disabilities

HEALTHY CHOICES

- Making choices
- Health relationships
- Skills for health

SUPPORT FOR HEALTH

- Individual basic needs
- Care
- Education
- Physical environment
- Economic change
- Rights and responsibilities
- Information

AIMS

- Reduce health inequalities
- Increase well-being
- Decrease disease, disability and avoidable deaths

PRINCIPLES

- The right to health and the right to understanding of health
- Equity in health
- Empowerment
- Community participation
- Partnership
- Accountability
- National and international co-operation

METHODS

- Community health development
- Education and training
- Planning
- Research and information

Figure 11.1   Model showing probable content of a proposed HS2000 Public Health Strategy Discussion Document.

Operational health promotion programmes

Both the health authority and the local authority's Health and Consumer Services Department decided in 1987 to move towards a programme style of management. Distinct and time-limited programmes of work were established

Table 11.2   Some HS2000 joint operational health promotion programmes (1990)

ESTABLISHED	Joint Food Programme Joint Smoking Programme Two independent community health initiatives

FOR LAUNCH	'Heart of Our City'
	    (Heart disease prevention programme)
	'Working for Health! Contracts'
	    (Work-place health programme)
	City-wide support for further independent community
	    health initiatives

BEING DEVELOPED	Joint Alcohol Programme Joint Accident Prevention Programme

for each major specific health topic, once the topic was endorsed by the parent organization as one of its priorities for action. In 1989 a smaller but important group of health promotion workers employed by or relating to the Family Practitioner Committee was also established, on much the same basis.

Since the earliest days of HS2000 there has been a vision of pooling these scarce human resources, so as to work in a co-ordinated way on topics such as healthy eating, smoking, heart disease and accident prevention. There is now good support for this co-ordinated approach to deal with a wide range of other health promotion issues.

Some major operational health promotion programmes that have been run, or are shortly anticipated to run under the HS2000 identity, are shown in Table 11.2. The consequences of the HS2000 framework in terms of operational programmes extend further than those shown, however. For example, for those programmes such as women's health or AIDS education and prevention, where the dominant investment has been by the health authority, there is still a degree of jointness in the approach to planning.

Organization of joint health promotion programmes

Having experimented with ways of managing the pooling of staff between the organizations, the main issues that have emerged include the impossibility of transferring the line management of either group of workers to the other's organization; and the differing pay structures which result in different conditions and levels of pay for essentially similar work, a factor which can be demotivating for one group of employees. Consequently we have arrived at a model of joint working, for example in the smoking and nutrition programmes, in which both health and local authorities have separate and clearly identifiable staff, who, however, communicate and share their work frequently. A lead officer is identified within one of the organizations who has the duty of co-ordination. The overall programme of work is jointly determined, and the steering and review of work is conducted by a small joint steering group. A programmes subcommittee of HS2000 oversees the total picture of joint operational programmes.

Three main sources of finance for health promotion programmes have been used. One is mainstream finance from the parent organizations. This funds the Health Promotion Units in the local and health authorities. The health authority has been able to increase its investment in mainstream funding in 1989 and 1990 and has demonstrated its commitment to health promotion by creating a new Director of Health Promotion post.

The second approach has been through joint finance applications to the Joint Consultative Committee. The criteria for eligibility for joint finance are complex, and somewhat uncertain in respect of health promotion. The funds are largely used for what is defined as personal social services, and for the care of clients who are the responsibility of both health and local authorities such as those with mental illness and mental handicap. The finance is temporary, grants being either non-recurrent, or recurrent with increasing contribution by the sponsoring organization. Therefore, short-term finite projects apart, success in a joint finance application still involves mainstream funding by one or other parent organization within a comparatively short time.

The third approach to funding has been to seek external funding for model projects in which the distinctive factor is the HS2000 context. One such application, for funding a major heart disease programme in which the intervention phase relies on collaboration between a wide range of health and local authority departments, has been successful. This appears largely to be because of the ability to demonstrate a well-advanced intent to deliver, which crosses organizational divides (covering education, recreation, social services, environmental health, primary care and hospitals).

The balance between strategic and operational energy

From the earliest vision of HS2000 there were those who wanted to develop health promotion topics, those who wanted to develop a health promotion strategy, and those who wanted to do both at the same time. Four years on, the choice does not appear any easier:

1 An investment solely in health topic based programmes would appear to be vulnerable to changes in organizational priorities, particularly at a time of financial stringency which can easily lead to marginalization of new initiatives.
2 A joint approach without sufficiently conspicuous programme activity can appear time-wasting and boring to practitioners and does not easily attract media coverage since there is nothing to portray with an immediate human dimension.

It seems that the ideal local strategy would be to have a mix of strategic and programme development, provided that there is enough in the way of financial and human resource to do both.

The nature of the work involved in the initiative of 1990

Human resources

There is still only one full-time post supporting the initiative, the HS2000 Co-ordinator. This post was jointly funded from 1988 with an increasing share of the funding now falling to the health authority. In addition 1.2 whole-time equivalents are contributed by Sheffield City Council for two part-time ad-ministrative and support posts.

The majority of those involved in the initiative are available for HS2000-related activities for only a small proportion of their time. This includes per-haps thirty health and local authority officers and practitioners who contribute four hours a week or less with the backing of their parent organizations.

Financial resources

The funding position is now complex, because of the different sources and time scales. The majority of the health programmes and other activity relat-ing to HS2000 are funded by the parent organizations and therefore do not appear as an identified budget relating to HS2000. A breakdown of the funding is shown in Table 11.3.

Activities

The nature of the activities that the core (and other) workers are currently involved in can be condensed into the following categories:

1 Developing, negotiating and producing the Sheffield strategy for Health for All.
2 Providing and exchanging information for health promotion planning and management purposes, between the major information sources in the city.
3 Designing and co-ordinating specific health promotion programmes.
4 Servicing and organizing the various committees and working groups.
5 Training on Health for All, and social marketing of the HS2000 initiative in a variety of sectors. It is intended to fund training and development posts so as to increase this effort. The aim will be to increase the effective-ness, and perceived relevance of the contacts with the city's academic institutions, with those City Council departments not so far active, with those parts of the health authority that do not yet see themselves as health promoters, with an ever-wider range of voluntary and community groups, with the professions and trade unions, and with a number of distinct commercial initiatives specific to Sheffield. These include the 1991 World Student Games organization and the various committees that link the local authority and commercial sectors with responsibility for planning large developments in the city.
6 Liaising with a number of relevant national organizations. These include the United Kingdom Healthy City Network, the Local Authority Health

Table 11.3   HS2000: main sources of health promotion funding 1989/90

Category of expenditure	Joint finance (£000s)		Mainstream (£000s)	
HS2000 Core	Main part of HS2000 Co-ordinator salary, and office costs	25.3	Balance of HS2000 Co-ordinator salary and support staff:	
			Health Authority	3.4
			City Council	14.2
HS2000 Health Promotion	Smoking Programme	15.3	Health Promotion	145.0
Programmes and Demonstration Projects			Centre (Health Authority)	
			Health Promotion and Research Unit (City Council)	198.8
Support for Independent Community Health Initiatives	Community Health Development Worker	17.5		
	Sharrow Community Health Project	12.3		
	Occupational Health Project/ Trade Union Safety Committee	37.0		
	Totals	107.4		361.4

Network, the Association of Metropolitan Authorities, the Health Education Authority, the Faculty of Public Health Medicine, the Institute of Health Service Management and the Institution of Environmental Health Officers. Much is also learned in exchanges with those workers in other cities, both in the UK and Europe that are involved in developing their own Healthy Cities.

In summary, and looking forward

In Sheffield the local approach to Health for All (based on thirty-eight ready-made European targets) that initially appeared so useful, has been dropped. The new strategy will give prominence to the original HFA principles, incorporated into a new conceptual framework. This promotes the major determinants of health and ill-health in a way that is locally agreed to be of concern. Creating targets, and indicators arising from these concepts, is the next step.

We found no solution to the choice of whether to invest money and energy either into strategic level work or into operational programmes. Both are clearly and urgently required for long term effectiveness.

HFA is not an easy commodity to market, to organizations or to the community. We plan now to achieve more penetration and more perceived relevance and involvement across the city.

The stage of organizational partnerships is partly achieved and underway. Partnership with the community appears a truly major and vital challenge. This is the next hurdle.

Acknowledgements

My most grateful thanks to our Healthy Sheffield 2000 Co-ordinator, Maddy Halliday, for major contributions both to the Initiative and to this chapter. There are many other closely involved colleagues, but I would like to single out and express my gratitude to Carol Thomas, formerly Health Promotion Research Officer, Sheffield Health Authority; Geoff Green, formerly Principal Officer, Central Policy Unit, Sheffield City Council; and John Rice, Assistant Director of Health and Consumer Services, Sheffield City Council and Chair of the HS2000 Planning Team in 1989/90.

References and further reading

Black Report (1980) *Inequalities in Health: Report of a Research Working Group*, London: Department of Health and Social Security.
Halliday, M. (1990) *Healthy Sheffield 2000 Annual Review 1989*, Healthy Sheffield 2000 Office, Sheffield City Council.
Sheffield Health Authority (1986) *Health Care and Disease: A Profile of Sheffield*, Departments of Community Medicine and Information, Sheffield Health Authority.
Thunhurst, C. (1985) *Poverty and Health in the City of Sheffield*, Health and Consumer Services Department, Sheffield City Council.

12

Horsens

*Knud Bragh-Matzon
and Flemming Holm*

A June 1990 kaleidoscope

Chop-chop-chop. . . . An export clerk from the local bank is letting the knife
dance on vegetables in the back of the Healthy City shop in Horsens, Denmark. He is helped by two unemployed people, who are also feeding the
Moulinex machine. They are selling Healthy City pitta sandwiches on the
square in front of the shop. These people include a teacher, a dentist, a nurse
and a managing director from the local rubber company. The customers are
23,000 visitors to Horsens this last week in June. They have come from all
over Denmark to show the spirit of sport, when it is not competitive – an
activity by amateurs, just for the fun of it. The whole city has been reorganized around the needs of its visitors and guests.

The Health Council of Horsens has produced posters and leaflets on the
issue of sport injuries; a flying squad of youngsters from the local schools and
trade unions are distributing them among the athletes. At the same time a
private dentist is using a lot of time trying to promote Horsens as the right
place for health education – Master of Public Health. The chairman of the
local general practitioners (GPs) are asking why so many health actions are
taking place, without their participation? Can we have a meeting about this?

Our board meets to discuss the budget: there are lots of problems. A liberal
politician starts chasing sponsors to support the Healthy City staffing and
activities.

The national television is telling the story of how senior citizens are
arranging alternative sports for one another. An army of white-haired people
play boccia and dance in the sports hall before noon, helping their colleagues
in wheelchairs living in residential homes to do the same!

Representatives from the city, the country, the priests, the hospital and the

GPs meet in the shop to create a prevention system for citizens with a personal crisis. Thirty-two self-help groups tackle cancer, divorce, child-terrorists, parent-terrorists, alcoholism and loneliness – all organized from the basement of the shop. For the first time we get the question in the shop: where do you report a company that is polluting the water?

This picture of June 1990 was part of our vision of health in Horsens when we first started thinking about it early in 1987. Even now we know it is only a step on the way; how can the vision be turned into reality?

Steps on the way from vision to reality

Ladies and gentlemen, where is health created? It is lived by people within the settings of their everyday life: where they learn, play, work, love. It is created in caring for yourself and others, in being able to take decisions and have control over one's life circumstances, in being assured that the society one lives in aims to create conditions that allow the attainment of health within that Society.

(Halfdan Mahler, former Director General of the World Health Organization, speaking at the Ottawa Conference, 1986)

This quotation specifies the most important preconditions for turning the vision of a Healthy City into reality. First of all it brings health far beyond the traditional health-sector and second (if you take it seriously), it gives a total new entry point to health. Health is not created in the health sector but it is created in our daily life, and is therefore a responsibility for all of us: politicians, professionals, economists, industrial managers, and so on.

This way of thinking is really the first step towards making the vision of health for all a reality. The basic understanding of the Healthy City Project as an all-embracing effort to look at health and not only disease, to look at all the powers influencing health, especially the positive ones, is essential and without doubt the most crucial point in building up a health promotion strategy. Mainly because this way of thinking moves the responsibility from traditional medical knowledge and activity to politics, leadership and management.

There are six important practical steps in the transforming process from vision to reality:

1 Political commitment and legitimacy.
2 Building up a small catalyst unit to secure the transformation process.
3 Building up an infrastructure to secure involvement and legitimation from the essential powers in city life.
4 Information, communication, visibility and public debates on health issues: bringing health high on the agenda of everyday life.
5 Combining short-term action and long-term planning.
6 Promoting and securing the process over time.

These six stages will now be discussed in turn.

Political commitment and legitimacy

A basic prerequisite to working with this holistic concept is the political acceptance and commitment of the City Council. This means that the top political level has to declare explicitly its support to the Health for All Strategy and the practical transformation process.

In other words, the City Council must be ready to involve ordinary citizens and other non-traditional partners and go beyond the traditional borders between professional and other sectors. It must also be ready to explore new and unknown paths – even paths that turn out to be wrong.

Without this political legitimation the necessary changes in the health system will be very hard to achieve. Securing this basic political engagement is a continuous process, not only in the starting phase, but also throughout the whole Healthy Cities Project.

Therefore, verbal commitment is not sufficient. You need an ongoing political debate on health issues, ideas about the Health for All vision in the practical world, and how as a politician I can secure their practical expression. This leads to the next basic step.

Building up a small catalyst unit to secure the transformation process

To transform the health promotion concept into praxis, it is necessary to build up a small flexible team to act as a catalyst or bridge between the existing system and the multiple powers and resources which exist in any city, even the poorest. One way to organize this is through creating a private foundation outside the city administration. This structure secures immediate action, separate from the municipal bureaucracy and provides a short cut between ideas and initiatives. Both are essential when working to achieve public involvement. In addition this approach is an advantage when it is a matter of breaking down traditional borders between different professions and sectors.

By providing a neutral ground where it is legitimate to seek new solutions to old, well-known problems, it is possible to move the focus from problems to possibilities. At the same time such an independent body demonstrates in a public and visible way that this project is for the whole city and not a new department inside the city administration. For this reason another important step in the process is not to link the project to any single sector; in Denmark initiatives of this kind would usually be linked to the social and health sector. To be effective, the group must be independent or at least linked directly to the Mayor's office.

Staffing in the catalyst unit: the Healthy City team

The main task for the unit is mediating in the open space between the citizens, organizations, private sector and the political/administrative level in the city. This demands a highly experienced interprofessional staff, with credibility and freedom to act and to use non-traditional methods without having to ask or seek permission when new steps need to be taken. In building up the team the following points should be noted:

1 It is a catalyst team and not a new department. Five or six people are the maximum staff; the task is to activate others.
2 Experienced and mainly senior staff are needed, probably taken from different sectors in the city administration and the manager of a team should perhaps be recruited among the chief officers in order to underline the importance of the team.
3 The staff should be drawn from different professional backgrounds to make explicit the holistic concept of the project.

Essential tools for the Healthy City team

1 The team needs very wide limits for action and initiatives and a budget sufficient to finance and see through good ideas immediately, e.g. buy project leaders out of their original job for shorter or longer periods.
2 The team must be allowed by the City Council to involve individuals from the city administration without permission in every case.
3 Lastly, the team needs the legitimacy to involve widely different organizations, companies, grass-roots individuals and others in the work.

This last condition needs a commitment beyond the political, and leads to the demand for a new infrastructure that involves a broader spectrum of partners from city life.

Building up an infrastructure to secure involvement and legitimation from the essential powers in city life

A major step in bringing the vision of a Healthy City into reality is the building up of a formal infrastructure to facilitate legitimacy of a broad approach to health work in the city. A structure that reflects the holistic approach and is in itself the mirror of the basic elements in the Health for All Strategy. In practice this means citizens in the steering committee and collaborating structures between sectors and professions that traditionally are not connected with health or working together.

One example is the infrastructure that has been built up in Horsens where the members of the Health Committee are politicians from the City and County Council, chief executives, trade unions, employers' organizations and ordinary citizens without links to any special organization or interest. The Committee is the overall steering group for the whole project and secures through its composition communication links between important 'health creators' in the city. The main task for the Committee is to create more effective links in health politics and planning. This is done in continuing planning meetings with participation from the professional group. Members of this group are professionals that, directly or indirectly, through their daily work are influencing the health conditions in the city.

The group includes not only traditional health workers, such as general practitioners, hospital doctors, dentists and nurses, but also private architects, police officers, planners, technicians, cultural and social workers. All in all about twenty different professions are represented and what is remarkable is that they are doing it on a voluntary basis. Besides participating in the overall planning process the group supervises the Healthy City team and other political and practical actions in the city.

An obvious task is of course to act as an interprofessional forum for new initiatives, methods and ideas. The two bodies together secure the common commitment and legitimation of the political/administrative level and of professionals and other important powers in daily city life. With these mechanisms in place, the framework for an overall approach exists.

Information, communication, visibility and public debates on health issues: bringing health high on the agenda of everyday life

To send the signal that the city takes the Health for All Strategy seriously, it is necessary to show the importance in a physical way. Therefore, a Healthy City Shop was opened in Horsens in the centre of the town where city life is lived. The shop is open to everyone and acts as the central point for health promotion development in the city. The shop is used by the Healthy City team, citizens, professionals, grass-roots initiatives and self-help groups. It has become an active communication and developing centre concerning health initiatives, debates, exhibitions and specific action.

It has become one of the most important and concrete steps towards realizing the vision, mainly because it gives the public the possibility of bringing its own visions about a Healthy City into reality through the support offered by the team in the shop. To a certain extent it has become the focal point for health in the city and in that sense the best communication source we have. It facilitates what we call 'positive rumours' among the citizens concerning their practical possibilities of influencing the health conditions of the city.

Working with the media

Another essential step is to work on a broader information scale than is traditionally done by the health sector. It is necessary first to inform the whole city about the Health for All vision, and second, to provide information on the practical outcomes of activities that are undertaken. One approach has been a periodical Healthy City newspaper delivered to every household in the city. More important has been the Healthy City magazine every second week on the local radio. Another entry-point is to involve the existing media – local and regional radio, television, and newspapers. Our concept has simply been to involve individual journalists, giving them the feeling of the potential in the strategy and of their own personal role as communicators and public health leaders. In this very simple way the interest of the media in health issues has increased and other themes have been gradually brought into the context of a Healthy City – not by us, but by the media themselves.

Combining short-term action and long-term planning

Turning visions into realities is hard work and needs an overall strategy with the basic idea of working on two parallel levels:

1 a short-term action-orientated level
2 a long-term planning level.

The main goal of the action-orientated level is the involvement and engagement of as many people and partners in the city as possible. This means in practice that it is essential that ideas and initiatives, no matter how small or unimportant they might seem, must be transformed into realities. In this context, it is not important that such initiatives may not have a major or even any impact on the existing systems. What really matters is their expression of engagement and commitment from citizens, professionals and institutions. Projects brought forward by interested people usually influence everyday life at a street level and therefore are more easily accepted by the population at large. In that sense they are the preconditions for a wider participation and in the end they provide a breeding ground for change. The work on the action level has to be seen from the point of view of process and not only from that of outcome and results. This approach is a key point in turning visions into realities. Ideas have to be enabled to materialize, especially aiming at public participation.

It is of extreme importance that every single project is built up and steered by a responsible group with representatives from the most different, but relevant, sectors, organizations and citizens. Moreover, this group should be built from motivated individuals rather than representatives from 'organized systems'. It is in this way that the first seeds for real intersectoral collaboration is created.

If this method is combined with more major initiatives started or brought forward by the Health Committee, professional group or others, the preconditions for reorienting the existing system can be brought about. This process is vital in the transformation of the health system, but it cannot be done without the parallel work on the more long-term planning level.

Politically this level is secured through the composition of the Health Committee, but in order to keep health on the agenda in important existing bodies, the manager of the Healthy City staff, for example, has a permanent seat in the overall planning group for the whole city. Through these continuing efforts to bring health aspects into the heart of city decisions, together with the concrete and visible projects, we have managed after two years to set Health for All as the main target for the overall city plan in Horsens. This historic decision in the city council commits all sectors not only to plan along the lines of Health for All, but actually to carry it out in practice.

Promoting and securing the process over time

To keep the political and professional commitment over the years, it is essential to have a set of base-line data as a starting-point for measuring the efforts towards a healthier city. To secure this base line, a national Health Survey Institute was engaged to carry out a health profile for us. The survey was done by interviewing around 1,000 citizens in their own homes.

Besides giving us a base line, it has given us a picture of the health situation in Horsens, not only through hard statistical data, but also in the way it is felt and perceived by the citizens themselves. In that sense it has given us an excellent basis for our work and an indispensable tool in the evaluation process that provides sustainable political support.

Finally, it is essential to underline that all the above mentioned should go together: it is not a step-by-step strategy. Maybe even more important: you should always be ready to change structures, methods and even thinking according to the experience you will inevitably gain, but of course without losing the basic ideas. What is needed is a flexible organic structure: a Healthy City project can never be stationary or bureaucratic. The goal is to provide a framework for people to act in and not to tell them what is good and what is not.

If we can manage that, the change to the better in everyday life will occur and the Healthy City vision can completely change urban reality and not only be an embellishment on the existing world.

A June 1990 postscript

After four fantastic days, 23,000 amateur athletes have left Horsens. A lot of injuries, in spite of the posters, a lot of parties in the street at night – lots of fun. In the back of the Healthy City shop sits the export clerk, wondering what went wrong: there wasn't a big market for healthy pittas. In fact our clerk and his crew from the Health Committee must face a minor deficit. The clerk shakes his head, but at the same moment the door bell rings and a group of citizens whom we have not seen before enter the shop saying, 'We just learned about the Healthy City idea on the radio, what about this idea we have had. . . .'

13

Gothenburg

Ingvar Svensson

Introduction

If you asked ordinary citizens in Gothenburg, Sweden, if our city is a healthy place in which to live, a frequent answer would be 'No'. If you continued and asked 'Why?', many people would refer to serious air pollution, periodic attacks of thermal inversion and similar environmental problems. Many people are frightened of the effects of these phenomena on their health and it is not unusual for people, who have the opportunity, to move out to the suburbs. However, when they return to the city, to work, or shop, or visit the theatre, they usually do so by car with the consequence that emissions from cars is now the city's worst source of pollution.

When we look at the statistics (Public Health Report 1 1987), there are health data which indicate that the situation in some respects is worse than either the general picture in Sweden or specifically that of other cities. However, there are also data which indicate a current trend towards a better level of health than we have ever had before in our city.

Gothenburg: a city based on industry

Gothenburg is a city of some 430,000 inhabitants; 34,000 are of pre-school age, younger than 6 years old, 50,000 are between 7 and 18 and 81,000 are older than 65 (18.8 per cent of the total). Compared with Sweden as a whole Gothenburg has fewer children of pre-school age and more pensioners. Altogether 280,000 people work in Gothenburg; the city itself is the largest employer with 70,000 employees (City Office 1990).

About 56,000 people are employed in the manufacturing industry and of these 70 per cent are working in engineering. Gothenburg and its region is Sweden's industrial centre with about one-quarter of the national capacity. The city is a centre for transport and has a large port. In the 1960s several of Sweden's largest shipyards were located here and employed a large share of the workforce but they have long since been closed. Consequently during the 1970s and 1980s there was a major restructuring of the labour market. During this restructuring of the local economy the registered unemployment was almost 4 per cent; by 1989 it had been reduced again to about 1.4 per cent (City Office 1990).

Swedish local government: the special position of Gothenburg

Sweden has two levels of local government, each enjoying considerable autonomy within a legislative framework and including the right to raise taxes for the services provided. These two levels are the counties (*landsting*) and within the counties the municipalities (*kommun*). In Sweden the munici- palities are responsible for among other things social services, schools, physi- cal planning and housing, environmental planning and control, water supply and refuse collection. The counties are responsible for health and medical services. Different laws regulate these responsibilities. The supreme governing body of the city is the City Council (*kommunfullmktige*), which consists of eighty-one politicians elected for a three-year period. Unusually in Sweden, the city of Gothenburg has the duties of both a municipality and a county. This dual role creates considerable opportunities to develop services to pro- mote public health.

The city government itself is engaged in many different service sectors and engages some 70,000 employees. These are employed under about fifty dif- ferent committees with departments of the City Council and nearly as many trading companies owned by the city as by private enterprises. These committees are elected by the City Council.

The Council in addition to setting the local tax level also decides the fees for different services. It determines the responsibilities of the different com- mittees where these are not regulated by national legislation and sets policy guidelines and allocates funds to the committees within the framework of the City Council budget. The Council also elects an Executive Committee (*kommunstyrelse*), which has to prepare proposals on strategic matters. The Executive Committee is responsible for financing and also supervising the work of the different committees.

The committees are politically responsible for the work of their depart- ments directly to the Council. There are a number of standing committees such as those responsible for medical services, environmental and health protection and physical planning which cover the whole city area. Social services, schools, leisure services and libraries are now organized by twenty- one district committees, as part of a new move towards decentralization. The committee for medical services directs and co-ordinates the work of seven subcommittees which run the two large hospitals and five primary health care districts respectively.

Origins of health promotion in Gothenburg

The Council decided in 1975 to set up a commission of inquiry into health promotion (*friskvardsberedningen*). The initiative came from the medical services committee, which had recognized that their services were preoccupied with sickness and injuries. It was realized that working with health problems would involve both the medical as well as many other committees. Therefore the committee proposed that the City Council should set up a commission on health promotion. In the terms of reference given to the commission it was stated that it should define health promotion, make an inventory of ongoing activities and propose goals and guidelines for health promotion. It should also specify strategic activities and priorities, work out a suitable division of labour between different committees and departments, and define the role of the Executive Committee.

The report of the Health Promotion Commission (1979) was entitled *The Health of the People in Gothenburg: Views and Proposals*. In the technical report prepared by the secretary for the Commission, a broad overview of different aspects and conditions of health was presented as indicated by the section titles:

'Health and medical development'
'What is health and illness?'
'Sickness and death'
'The individual and society'
'Health care from the point of view of medical care'
'The condition of health in different environments'
'Health promotion'
'Environmental health'

The Health Promotion Commission stated that it had not scrutinized the secretary's report in detail but it supported the basic set of values underpinning it, the general views expressed and guidelines proposed in it.

The report proposed that the Council should adopt the proposals as guidance for health promotion. It also proposed that the Council should draw the citizen's attention to the risks of abuse of alcohol, drugs and other such substances, and in particular that young people should abstain from their use.

The Council was also recommended to set up a standing Public Health Council (*Hlsordet*), consisting of two members elected from each of the leisure services committee, the environmental and health protection committee, the medical services committee, the schools committee and the social services committee.

The report proposed that the Public Health Council should work out guidelines for locally co-ordinated health promotion activities, encourage experimental work, arrange information and other activities against abuse, determine how to strengthen educational activities for parents and develop other activities which would increase the understanding of children's and young people's development and living conditions.

The Council was further recommended to take initiatives to put pressure on the national government to take action on the need for good housing for people living in modest circumstances and to guarantee that young people leaving school should be able either to find work or continue in further education.

The report was circulated to the various committees for comments. The general view was that the report was valuable, but many committees also asked for more concrete guidelines and detailed descriptions of what should be done.

The subsequent proposal from the executive committee, which was adopted by the City Council, addressed organizational matters, the delineation of the field of health promotion, goals and guidelines, strategic areas of activity and local experimental work. The Council voted for a small fund for the administrative costs of the Public Health Council during its start-up year.

The role of the Public Health Council was formally approved as the following (Report from Health Promotion Commission of Gothenburg 1981):

1 To direct and co-ordinate public health, based on a further evaluation of the report of the Commission and to develop programmes of activity (a programme against alcohol abuse had meanwhile been proposed by an ad hoc committee appointed by the Executive Committee).
2 To co-ordinate activities to build up a body of information about the public's state of health and health risks, and find ways to channel such information to those involved in health promotion.
3 To support contacts with academic and research bodies in respect of research and development work.
4 To take part in the Executive Committee's preparation of budgets and plans for the City Council's different committees and departments.

The Executive Committee proposed that members of the Public Health Council would be appointed by the committee itself and be chaired by a member of the Executive Committee. (As the Commission had proposed, its members should also be members of the other standing committees.)

The delineation of health promotion was another question for the Executive Committee. It was observed that the terms 'health' and 'health promotion' were used in many different ways. The Executive Committee defined its own use of the term 'health promotion' in the following way (Report from Health Promotion Commission of Gothenburg 1981):

Health promotion consists of activities having as the main purpose

- to identify conditions which, if no measures were taken, would lead to illness or injury or make it difficult for the individual to live in good health in the future

- to act against such conditions
- to support and facilitate the early discovery of symptoms.

The goals for health promotion were stated as follows:

Health promotion should support good health for the entire population. It should support the individual to protect, develop and take responsibility for his or her own health. Health promotion activities should be carried out with respect for the individual's integrity.
Health promotion should promote:

- a physical environment, which does not expose the individual to unnecessary risks, and a social environment, which promotes the individual's development, and provides support to protect the individual's health
- possibilities for individuals to promote their own health in daily life
- possibility of screening and other preventive activities through the medical services.

(Report from Health Promotion Commission of Gothenburg 1981)

When discussing strategic areas, two aspects were raised. First, the health problems focused on should be valid for large population groups or groups easy to identify. Second, it should be plausible that health promotion activities could affect health. Some areas were highlighted to be scrutinized first for programme work. These were environmental protection, conditions for growth and development of children and teenagers, problems of family living, tobacco, nutrition, physical activity and health education. The Public Health Council was also given the task of initiating experimental work to give more experience of how to organize and develop local health activities.

The Public Health Council established 1981

The Public Health Council was established in 1981 and was given the tasks mentioned above. Furthermore it was given the task of implementing the existing ad hoc programme against alcohol abuse. In reality during the early years this became the dominant part of its activity. The Executive Committee created a special fund of SKr 30 million (US$ 5 million), to be used for this purpose during a three-year period. This fund was used to support activities of both the standing committee and outside organizations engaged in this work. Information, education and alcohol-free public events for young people were the main areas of activity.

The council convened a group of experts, drawn from different departments, to work out a programme for health promotion. As a part of this programme experimental work was begun in one district. People from primary health care were involved as well as from leisure services, schools and social services. The participants were involved in both joint activities and in developing their own work at the primary health care centres and in the community. The experiences from this work showed that health promotion activities could be carried out only with engaged and competent personnel who could make health questions interesting to the general public.

Working out an overall programme for health promotion was a difficult task to achieve because of widely different opinions about priorities and the right way to proceed. To make further progress it was decided to invite an outside social medical consultant (Svärdsudd n.d.) to work through the background material prepared for the Health Promotion Commission and to bring it up to date. In his report to the Public Health Council he discussed the choice between preventive actions directed towards individuals with high risks and prevention aimed at the total population. It was concluded that a combination of a 'population' strategy and a 'high risks' strategy would be most likely to give the best preventive results.

The recommendations of this report to the council were that it should introduce action to

1 decrease tobacco-smoking, principally among young people
2 improve nutrition and dietary habits
3 reduce accidents
4 decrease alcohol abuse
5 stimulate physical activity in the general population
6 improve the psychosocial environment for socially and psychologically depressed groups.

This was the priority list. The intention had been to weigh the various possibilities to take action and achieve effect. It was argued that actions which can affect the health of a large group of people and have effects early in life should be given priority.

The proposed list of actions was accepted by the Public Health Council in 1983 and the city administrative office was instructed to work out action programmes for each of the topics, except for alcohol abuse where the existing programmes was judged to be sufficient. In addition the council added 'sexual relations' to the list because of the high incidence of abortion among teenagers and those in their early twenties in the city. It was also noted that the committee for environmental and health protection and its office had started to work out programmes for air, water and soil and concluded that an initiative from the Public Health Council was not needed. The health promotion programme was finally adopted by the City Council in spring 1985.

During most of the period 1981–5 the council had been supported by three technical groups (health promotion, alcohol and drugs). These groups involved experts from different departments. The chairman and the secretary came from the Executive Committee's staff. There was a lot of discussion with the department heads about the status of the groups and the experts' relations with their own departments, as those questions were seen as rather unclear. The experts themselves were also questioning their role. It therefore became necessary to reorganize the technical groups to be the major instrument for involving the departments in the implementation of the health promotion programme.

The health promotion programme (adopted 1985)

The programme consisted of goals and guidelines for each of the priority themes. As a general background and principle, it was stated that preventive work must start from the point of view of the people, their needs and their resources. The City Council believes that the individual is capable of creating his or her own consciousness of health and can take responsibility for it. At the same time it is important to disseminate knowledge (within the medical services and elsewhere) in such a way that an individual can take it, value it and use it. Different committees were given the task of carrying out the programme. They were encouraged to act together and to invite and support voluntary associations of different kinds in taking part.

As mentioned previously, Gothenburg is both a municipality and a county. The normal situation in Sweden is that health promotion programmes are worked out as a part of the counties' tasks in the field of medical services. These programmes are often carried out as a part of primary health care in co-operation with the different municipalities and their organization of committees and departments. The decision by the Council was to give the task of implementing the various programmes to different committees and departments depending on how the health promotion programme activities could be incorporated into their main tasks and strengthen their quality.

The example of nutrition is illustrative. The programme for nutrition stresses the importance of information and education to different key-groups, especially children and their parents and those engaged in the different service sectors who support them. Children's day-care centres and schools are important. The children eat there and nutrition habits are influenced by their experiences. Even if other groups can be reached by other activities in the programme, the way it is carried out in the schools is very important. The task of directing and co-ordinating the nutrition programme was therefore given to the school committee.

Responsibility for the other programmes was allocated in the following way:

Programme	*Committee*
tobacco	medical services
physical activity	leisure activities
accidents	environmental and health protection
psychosocial environmental	social services
sexual relations	schools

The Public Health Council had to follow, support and evaluate the implementation of the programme. The council was given a fund of SKr2 million (US$350,000) to support the activities.

During the years since 1985, the committees have had great freedom to find the best ways and activities to reach the population. For example, two of them, the nutrition programme and the sexual relations programme, have been very much engaged in educational activities. They have had courses for different personnel groups about how in their normal work they can bring out the health aspects in more effective ways.

Another programme on the psychosocial environment has, among other things, supported with advice and money a group of divorced men, whose children are living with their mothers; they have organized what is called 'the Sunday-fathers' club'. This now has over 300 members and has an important role for its members as a self-help group. It also arranges activities for the fathers and their children during summer holidays and week-ends. This club has also been very active in helping groups of divorced men both in other cities and in the Nordic countries to organize themselves.

The Public Health Council receives yearly reports from the committees on their work. The Council has also supported common activities, such as participation in exhibitions and fairs, which are visited by many people. An experience from these occasions was the somewhat unexpected effect of the absence of a regular specific project against alcohol abuse. Many committees were engaged in that work but there was no designated group with the task of co-ordination. The project leaders of the other projects made it clear that when talking about health-risks to the public at such events it was not possible to avoid talking about the use of alcohol. As a result, a special project was established.

When HIV-infection became obvious as a health problem the Executive Committee ordered the Public Health Council to be the steering-group at the political level for a co-ordinated action by the city administration. This work has included taking an overview of existing programmes and activities in the fields of protection against infectious diseases, prevention and care of drug abusers, counselling bureaux for young people and support for gay associations.

Other activities from the Public Health Council include a programme for asthma and allergy, a programme for a better social environment for young people in the central part of the city, and an evaluation of the alcohol programme. The council has also worked with other social organizations (the Church, Rotary Club, trade unions, the local branch of the International Organization of Good Templars and others) to establish a Foundation with the goal of finding new ways to work against drug abuse (*Stiftelsen for narkotikafritt Goteborg*).

The administrative culture in the city is now one of decentralization. This means among other things that the City Council is committed to adopting general goals and guidelines. The different committees then have to work out more concrete goals and strategies so that they can follow these guidelines in the best way within their funds. This also means that much co-ordinating work must be done on different levels, both by managers and by their subordinates especially at local level.

Several of the most important committees have been represented through their chairperson and vice-chairperson in the Public Health Council. But it was also decided that to be most effective the managers should be represented in a technical advisory group to the council. This group had previously consisted of experts of uncertain status. Now the members of this group are appointed by their managers with the explicit task of representing them at the meetings and regularly reporting back. As a result of this the people working in different activities initiated by the Public Health Council now feel that their work has the support of the top level within their organizations.

Reports on the state of the public health

Another initiative from the council during this period has been to establish an expert group with members both from the various departments, the University of Gothenburg and the Nordic School of Public Health. The task of this group is to analyse the state of health of the population. To date, two reports have been published. The first concentrated on the period 1975 to 1985 and was published in 1987. The second in 1989 presented a more in-depth picture of certain aspects noticed in the first report.

One such issue was the relationship between ill health and social problems. A high level of consumption of medical care was found in areas with many social problems. The connections between them are complex. The group used a case analysis approach to illustrate some particular risk-groups: people out of work, people living alone, immigrant women and children in multi-problem families. There are common aspects to these living conditions: problems in obtaining and keeping a job and problems in family relationships, both between the adults and between parents and children. There are also conflicts with other people in their social networks. These problems seem to be more frequent in these groups or at least are more regularly observed by the agencies with which they are in contact.

The expert group not only describes and analyses the problems, but also brings into the discussion ways to tackle them. It then becomes a task for the council to propose priorities and strategies following a public debate.

The group is currently preparing a report on the health of children and young people (Public Health Report 3 1991) and another report in which the existing statistical data are being analysed according to the twenty-one new neighbourhood districts. This will enable every district committee to have a report on the health situation in its area.

Gothenburg: a member of the WHO Healthy City Project

The Healthy City movement reflecting the concept of health promotion developed in the Ottawa Charter (WHO *et al.* 1986) and other WHO policy documents has brought us back to the prerequisites of health which were discussed at the starting-point of the development of health promotion in Gothenburg. We have engaged different sectors of the municipality's services in our health promotion programme. The Healthy Cities Project focuses in a distinct way on the reality that health problems can be handled in depth only through the engagement of the total urban society.

Co-operation and co-ordination with other cities in the WHO project has obliged us to scrutinize our programmes and efforts enabling us to search for better ways to engage different sectors and groups in our city. Our projects have in many ways achieved good results but only in limited areas of the health field and we have not yet reached a large proportion of the population. This was in one way an intended development of the different health promotion projects. During the early years they were seen as experimental work to develop models of good practice in their respective fields. When Gothenburg became involved with the WHO Healthy Cities Project it was time to start an evaluation of what had already been done.

However, going into the project also meant a challenge to deepen our view of health problems, which had started with the public health reports, but which had brought into focus the deeper physical, social and psychological dimensions of health in city life. One conclusion was that we now had to build up a number of complementary projects and activities, for example to promote health in working life. As a result of recognizing this, a health promotion project for employees in three of the City Council's own departments has been started and has inspired several more departments, who are now planning their own projects. A new impetus has also been given to implementing the promotion of health in socially and physically depressed areas of the city.

While this has been going on, there has been a large organizational change taking place in the city administration with the establishment of the twenty-one district committees and an emphasis on decentralization. As a direct result responsibility for several of the projects has been transferred to these district committees. They have been challenged to establish models of good health promotion in their day-to-day work which other district committees can then follow. This has also meant that the technical groups have now changed membership so that the staff of district departments are included.

Some experiences and reflections

As will be clear from this account, the process of developing a framework and models for the city's engagement in public health has been a continuing one over more than a decade. There have been both ups and downs. There have been both politicians and officials who have advocated this development in a very sensible and positive way. They have shown great awareness of the existing health problems and the prerequisites for health and they have supported the experimental work which has been necessary to develop health promotion. But of course the projects have also met people who have been more sceptical and generally uncommitted.

Some areas of positive development can already be identified. For example the Gothenburg health promotion projects have generated knowledge and activities in a way that has engaged people who are not normally reached by media coverage advertisment of healthy lifestyles even when the projects have been on a relatively small scale. They have also, by activities designed to influence and support routine municipal services, laid a foundation for further development. During the last year we have noticed that various committees have started their own health promotion programmes and demanded support, money and advice from the Public Health Council both for their own activities and for use in co-operation with voluntary organizations. For example the medical services committee supported several voluntary organizations in the preparation and distribution of a study-book on health promotion (Medical Services Committee 1990). Several of the new district committees have started their work inviting their population to become involved in new activities in health-promotion, thereby showing that the district committee reform also means to carry out new integrated forms of activities.

Another area to mention is the ongoing work to deepen knowledge and understanding of existing health problems which has been made possible by the series of public health reports (Public Health Reports 1987; 1989; 1991). These have been received with interest both by citizens and from the political and administrative bodies of the city. However, there is still much more to do to bring the reports into the centre of public debate.

What have been the prerequisites for this positive development and what lessons do they have for the future? Three main points stand out:

1 Personnel involved in the projects should be committed to their tasks, have good knowledge of their respective fields and also have an understanding of the different groups' total needs.
2 There should be explicit political aims and guidelines and a continuing interest by the Public Health Council and by the committees of the City Council in what is happening in the projects and how they reach out and affect public health.
3 It is absolutely necessary to have the interest and support from top management in the relevant departments.

At the same time there have been obstacles. It has not always been in every case an easy task to secure the broad engagement of the departments concerned. Preventive work has to struggle against what are perceived as the main tasks for the departments when it comes to claims on the budget and managerial support. Acute medicine, social services and care of children and the elderly population are generally seen as much more in the mainstream of interest and priority. Even when people realize the value of preventive work it is in reality a large step from that understanding to significant changes in the use of resources. This point is in fact underlined by the dramatic exception in the case of HIV/AIDS, where there have been significant changes both in interest and support from those parts of the municipal services which have been involved in allocating funds.

One dilemma which those supporting health promotion have met is that of measuring activities and results. The traditional services are well-known and there are usually known standards and ways of describing the work which has been done (albeit not always very well). One can notice that one of the main purposes of health promotion is to influence the standards of those services in ways that will change their qualities by giving them new aims and new contents.

For both supporters and those hesitating, the way to resolve this is by requesting evaluation studies for both traditional services and health promotion innovations.

The lack of such studies is often a drawback but in the short run we can derive support by working in areas of significance for health promotion. We are dealing with the known effects of tobacco, alcohol and drugs and observing that people's continuing interest in participating in different activities and also participation in such activities by people not so engaged before can be used as acceptable methods for evaluating the short-term results of these projects.

Another dilemma facing health promotion is the intense discussion about environmental problems. These arouse much interest and debate and we must address these issues if we are to reach the objective of a sustainable world. Large investments in environmental control and structural changes in the economy are necessary for reaching such an aim. However, from our public health reports we can see that the other obstacles to improved public health are primarily lifestyle and social conditions and this places a focus on the individual, the family and the social environment and both lifestyle and environmental issues must be addressed in parallel.

The final problem is to identify and bring order into describing what are the conditions for public health. Our health reports are rather good at identifying groups and areas with significant health problems and when showing significant differences between our city and other parts of the country. It is much more difficult to get straight answers about the reasons for the phenomena and to arrive at a consensus among researchers. This means that it is necessary to continue to argue for the value of preventive work and to meet the objections which are proposed. Such argument places health promotion in the mainstream of political debate and that is a very necessary step forward.

References

City Office (1990) *Statistical Yearbook Gothenburg 1990*. (Göteborgs Stadskansli 1990. *Statistisk årsbok Göteborg 1990*.) Gothenburg: Healthy Cities Project, City Office.

Medical Services Committee (1990) *Feel Well in Gothenburg*. (Göteborgs Sjukvård 1990. *Må bra i Göteborg*.) Gothenburg: Healthy Cities Project, City Office.

Public Health Report 1 (1987) *Development of Health in Gothenburg 1970–85.* (Hälsorådet i Göteborg 1987. Folkhälsorapport 1. *Folkhälsoutvecklingen i Göteborg 1970–85.*) Gothenburg, Healthy Cities Project, City Office.

Public Health Report 2 (1989) (Hälsorådet i Göteborg 1989. Folkhälsorapport 2.) Gothenburg: Healthy Cities Project, City Office.

Public Health Report 3 (1991) *Health of Children and Young People.* (Hälsorådet i Göteborg 1991. Folkhälsorapport 3. *Barns och ungdomars hälsa.*) Gothenburg: Healthy Cities Project, City Office.

Report from Health Promotion Commission of Gothenburg (1979) *Proceedings from City Council of Gothenburg* no. 223A. (Göteborgs Kommunfullmäktiges handlingar 1979. *Rapport från kommunfullmäktiges friskvårdsberedning* nr 223A.) Gothenburg: Healthy Cities Project, City Office.

Report from Health Promotion Commission of Gothenburg (1981) *Proceedings from City Council of Gothenburg* no. 176. (Göteborgs Kommunfullmäktiges handlingar 1981.) Gothenburg: Healthy Cities Project, City Office.

Svärdsudd, K. (no date) *Evaluation of Proposal on Health Promotion Program.* (*Utvärdering av förslag till friskvårdsprogram.*) Mimeo. Gothenburg: Healthy Cities Project, City Office.

WHO, Health and Welfare Canada, Canadian Public Health Association (1986) *Ottawa Charter for Health Promotion*, Copenhagen: WHO.

14

Eindhoven

Jan van der Kamp and
Janine Cosijn

Introduction

Eindhoven is located in the south-east of The Netherlands and is one of the oldest cities. It was granted a royal charter in 1232. Until the late sixteenth century it was a market and fortress town with a castle, walls and moats. As a result of fires and wars, little remains of this past.

Nowadays Eindhoven and its surroundings form the high-tech centre of The Netherlands with approximately 500,000 inhabitants. The city of Eindhoven was formed by a merging of five small villages and now has a population of approximately 200,000 inhabitants. It is an industrial heartland where electronics and related industries obviously play an important role. Countless companies in a variety of sectors are at home in Eindhoven. Its favourable location is an important factor in the town's pivotal position. The international ports of Antwerp and Rotterdam and cities such as Amsterdam, Brussels, Liège, Cologne and Düsseldorf are each approximately one hundred kilometres away.

Eindhoven's central position in industry, trade and science means that a great wealth of knowledge is available. That knowledge is transferred in various forms of co-operation between industry and educational institutes such as the Eindhoven University of Technology and the Eindhoven Polytechnic.

In a tourists' brochure Eindhoven is also described as a pleasant city to live in. The municipality is working hard on urban renewal. Many houses are newly built or renovated. Public parks, recreation grounds and children's playgrounds are spread all over the city. Eindhoven aims to create a healthy environment for all its citizens. In 1987 Eindhoven was the first winner of the National Environment Award.

All this and other health promotion initiatives were important elements for WHO to nominate Eindhoven as project city in its Healthy Cities Project.

A strategy for health promotion

An impulse to innovate public health in The Netherlands has existed for a considerable period. In 1986, the thirty-eight European Targets for Health for All of WHO were translated into a national health policy memorandum, called 'Nota 2000' (WVC 1986). In this document the national government expresses the shift from a health care policy towards a healthy public policy.

In Eindhoven the local health policy is based on this national health policy. In 1987 a charter was written which was meant to be an elaboration of this Nota 2000 with regard to a prevention policy and more specifically with regard to health promotion at the local level (van der Kamp and Cosijn 1987). This charter was accepted by the City Council of Eindhoven as a total vision of the Municipal Public Health Services' course to follow for the next years.

With regard to health promotion in Eindhoven, a 'structure-follow-strategy' approach was chosen. This strategy is concerned with creating possibilities for innovations in content. The strategy in Eindhoven is to stimulate innovations that link up with the ecological view of health. Marketing techniques have proved to be very effective for this workstyle.

In the classical health education approach, 'selling' a message is a central principle, in spite of all efforts made to take the potential customers into account. In this approach interventions are planned as isolated projects.

The changed view of health (a state of complete physical, social and mental well-being instead of merely the absence of disease) and the possibilities of the use of new techniques have created many opportunities to increase the effectiveness of health promotion.

Health promotion activities can be formulated in terms of a 'buyer's market'. Providing service is therefore a key element of health promotion in Eindhoven. Making use of potential buying processes has proved to be very effective. It also has an extra advantage: a more constructive realization of intersectoral action for the benefit of health becomes possible. The key element of this strategy is that the other is no longer considered to be an opponent with whom a conflict has to be solved, but that the other is an equal partner with whom a common goal – improving people's health – can be set and solved.

Health promotion in Eindhoven

In 1988, when Eindhoven joined the international Healthy Cities Project, the municipality had just changed its political and bureaucratic organization. As a consequence of this municipal reorganization, ad hoc structures such as for a special Healthy Cities Project Office are not allowed. Health promotion and Healthy Cities initiatives have to fit in the overall municipal health policy. Therefore Eindhoven has no separate Healthy Cities Office, but is carrying out its functions by means of the Health Promotion Department of the Municipal Public Health Services.

In this new municipal organization, the executive municipal services – such as the Municipal Public Health Services – are responsible for designing municipal policy. The executive services have to develop policy propositions in close collaboration with private organizations and community representatives. This approach stimulates intersectoral action based on equity between all organizations, groups and individual citizens involved.

The Health Promotion Department of the Municipal Public Health Services is responsible for initiating, stimulating and helping to realize health promotion within municipal policy. In the past few years several initiatives based on the principles of health promotion as stated in the Ottawa Charter were started. The three selected examples show a positive approach in enabling people to increase their control over their own health, their lifestyle and their environment.

An information centre on health

The first result of working on an ecological strategy for health promotion together with using marketing techniques was a public information centre for health: the *Gezondheidswijzer*. This centre started in 1984 from the assumption that people have an active role in gathering information on behalf of their own health, in the same way as if they are shopping in a supermarket.

In the *Gezondheidswijzer* – a kind of health information shop – everybody can obtain information on health, healthy lifestyles and coping with illness and disease. The main objective of the *Gezondheidswijzer* is to offer comprehensible information on health:

1 to improve people's ability to deal with health (problems) themselves
2 to enable people to share responsibility for their own and each other's health
3 to increase the emancipation of patients
4 to stimulate and support self-help and lay care initiatives.

The most important task of the *Gezondheidswijzer* is to make this information accessible for everyone. The selection of written material is based on criteria of comprehensibility for people who have no medical knowledge or background. The centre possesses the following materials: addresses of many local, regional and national health care organizations, patients' associations and self-help groups; written information such as magazine and newspaper articles, leaflets and brochures and a small library with reference books. Photocopies can be made of literature or articles. Leaflets and brochures are sold if they are not free of charge. No materials are lent out. In response to any question by mail, telephone or personal contact, the appropriate information will be supplied.

Besides the normal supply of information, the *Gezondheidswijzer* also has a 'weekly special'. All information on one special subject is offered free of charge during the week; the weekly subjects are announced by local radio and by local newspaper. The supply of information is under the full responsibility of the Municipal Public Health Services but no medical advice or consultation is given at the centre.

The *Gezondheidswijzer* started as a joint initiative of the Women's Council in Eindhoven and the Municipal Public Health Services. The centre is staffed by volunteers, all of whom are women. It has been agreed that the Women's Council of Eindhoven takes care of the daily organization and the selection and training of the volunteers. These volunteers generally have different tasks such as checking and keeping up the address files, the check and supply of brochures, the gathering and documentation of articles. In view of the yearly increase of the workload of these volunteers since the start of the information centre, the appointment of a professional co-ordinator has become essential for the future.

The *Gezondheidswijzer* appears to be successful in meeting needs, considering the growing number of requests. There is an average increase of clients of 30 per cent a year. There were 800 clients in the first year and 1,200 in the second. In 1989, more than 5,000 people asked for information at the centre.

Within the last three years, two more Public Health Services in the surrounding areas of Eindhoven have opened information centres on health working under the same name *Gezondheidswijzer* and on the same principles as in Eindhoven. The Association of Public Health Services in The Netherlands considers these public information centres on health an important element of health promotion and is therefore stimulating the creation of a network of these information centres all over the country.

Eindhoven's policy on lay care initiatives

In a similar way, support for self-help groups in Eindhoven was started. The City Council had many requests for financial support of lay care initiatives such as self-help groups. Not knowing exactly how to handle this kind of community health initiative, the City Council charged the Municipal Public Health Services to prepare a policy document on lay care. In 1985 this policy document was accepted by the City Council of Eindhoven (van der Kamp 1985).

Lay care refers to all health care given by lay people to each other in both natural and organized settings and by individuals themselves (Kickbusch and Hatch 1983).

In the Eindhoven policy document on lay care, four major types of lay care were distinguished:

1 Individual self-care which refers to unorganized health activities and health-related decision making by individuals. It encompasses self-treatment and self-medication.
2 Mutual care which refers to forms of spontaneous lay help that are provided by family, neighbours, friends, etc.
3 Volunteer care which is lay care provided by community members, but organized by agencies such as the church and voluntary associations.
4 Self-help groups which are groups of fellow sufferers concerned with common problems (van Harberden and Lafaille 1979). Self-help groups form around very specific and concrete problems. The distress experienced is mainly of a non-material and psychosocial nature. Although numerous self-help groups form around a disease or handicap, this disease or handicap never stands alone: with self-help groups it is always connected with psychosocial factors such as loneliness, fear, lack of understanding and stigmatization. In self-help groups, fellow sufferers learn from each other's experiences and from each other's knowledge. This knowledge comes from experience rather than from books or from the conventional 'authoritative' detached knowledge of experts.

Enabling people to take their own responsibility regarding their health and making individuals less dependent on professional care are central themes in Eindhoven's policy on lay care. The operationalization of this policy is realized in different ways.

Individual self-care is promoted through the health education programmes in schools. The *Gezondheidswijzer* plays a very important role in providing information on self-care activities.

Mutual and volunteer care activities are often supported by the health education officers working at the Municipal Public Health Services and the Local District Nursing Services. These health education officers organized, for example, courses on the practical and emotional aspects of home nursing by lay people.

Several self-help groups in Eindhoven are supported in a facilitating way by the Municipal Public Health Services. This support consists of a support in kind. Conference and meeting space is made available for these groups, as well as copying and mailing facilities. Educational materials are available for free. Groups are supported in getting started, in organizing meetings and with their public relations such as leaflets, brochures, posters, newsletters, and so on.

In the second stage of policy operationalization and implementation, the local authorities in Eindhoven should, according to the lay care policy document, actively participate in deliberations and consultations between the self-help and lay care groups and those organizations and institutions which might help to realize the objectives of these groups.

Another task of the local authorities is to approach private enterprises and initiatives such as health insurance companies to support self-help and lay care efforts in a more structured way. The elaboration of this advocacy function of the Municipal Public Health Services to increase the awareness of other professional care organizations and institutions with regard to their role in supporting community health initiatives, has started recently.

The Environment Project

In 1987 the City of Eindhoven launched a special programme for the prevention of minor vandalism in one specific neighbourhood in Eindhoven. This neighbourhood is the most recently built, in which the latest developments in the field of town planning and architecture have been put into practice. There are many young families with very young children. When compared with other areas in Eindhoven, there does not yet seem to be a lot of crime. But, in the next few years the number of inhabitants will increase and in order to maintain the present living conditions, crime prevention seems to be necessary. Therefore the City of Eindhoven considers not only the control of petty crime to be important, but also the prevention of it. An intersectoral municipal committee on the prevention of minor vandalism found several possible solutions for this problem, one of them being a special project for the children of the local primary schools.

The main objective of the 'Environment Project' was to teach the children to add line and meaning to their lives by means of a set of lessons which were 'tailormade' to their situation. With the help of these lessons they could explore their environment and become more familiar with it.

By means of this set of lessons the children are taught to accept more responsibility for their own environment. In learning this, it is hoped that they will absorb automatically the values and rules of society. And in this way, instead of being confronted with a prohibition of graffiti, they might consider damaging bus shelters as something that is not done.

The project, co-ordinated by the Health Promotion Department of the Municipal Public Health Services, started in 1988. Primary schools in the neighbourhood were asked if they were interested in lessons set for their pupils aimed at discovering their own environment; lessons which directly referred to the neighbourhood in Eindhoven where these children lived. After the project was explained, all schools agreed to participate.

The project started with a questionnaire based on the Seattle KidsPlace principle (Mayor's Survey 1984): asking how children experience their own living conditions and especially what they consider to be positive and negative in them. The overall impressions of the 10-year-old children in this specific neighbourhood in Eindhoven were positive: it is a clean, quiet, wonderful place to live in. Many children praised the facilities for playing outside; the presence of other children to play with was especially appreciated. A little more than 50 per cent of the children admitted minor vandalism once in a while, but more than 85 per cent thought vandalism to be annoying. Dog-dirt and traffic were considered to be the most important problems for these children.

The results of this inquiry formed the starting point for a set of lessons which were presented in January 1989 to those children who had filled in the questionnaire. The lessons were designed by the Environmental Education Centre in Eindhoven, The Netherlands Road Safety Association, the Education Faculty of the Tilburg Polytechnic and the Health Promotion Department of the Municipal Public Health Services. The lessons were edited by the municipal intersectoral committee for the prevention of minor vandalism in Eindhoven. The lessons were directly designed for the children living in this specific area of Eindhoven. With the help of a detailed map of their neighbourhood, they could indicate their own homes, the homes of their friends, their schools, and so on. Photographs used in the set could be recognized as taken in their own shopping centres and their own playgrounds.

An important characteristic of these lessons was that the chosen methods referred to the development of personal skills such as: enhancing problem-solving capacities; learning to make choices; learning to think critically; learning responsibility; managing socially. The lessons were not imposed by the teachers. The teachers and the children were invited to work with them. The schools who worked with the set lessons were enthusiastic. The lessons have an attractive presentation, because every situation can be recognized. The children enjoyed working with the lessons. The different assignments could be realized very well, although they sometimes took much time.

Until now, only the set lessons have been evaluated. The evaluation of the main objective of this project: learning to be responsible for your own environment, your own neighbourhood, has not been carried out yet.

Conclusion

The health promotion activities described are a selection of initiatives to make Eindhoven a healthy city. People are enabled to take control over the health aspects of their lives by following the current do-it-yourself trend in our Western society. People want to organize their own lives. They want to be more independent of structures and systems; they want to develop more initiatives and carry more responsibilities themselves.

Health promotion creates conditions respecting people's needs with regard to the development of their own skills in respect to health. Offering service and facilitating community health initiatives by enabling, mediating and advocacy functions, is therefore considered one of the major tasks of the local authorities i.e. the Health Promotion Department of the Municipal Public Health Services in Eindhoven.

References and further reading

Cosijn, J. (1989) *Supporting Lay Care: A Municipal Policy in Eindhoven*, Paper prepared for the fourth Healthy Cities Symposium in Pècs (Hungary), Eindhoven: Municipal Public Health Services.

Cosijn, J. (1991) 'Lokale gezondheidsinitiatieven en de rol van de gemeente', in E. de Leeuw (ed.), *Gezonde Steden* (in press).

Cosijn, J. and Leeuw, E. de (1991) *The Netherlands Healthy Cities Network Newsletter, Special edition 1991*. Eindhoven: Netwerk Gezonde Steden.

Davidson, E. (1989) *The Health Information Centre in Eindhoven*, Paper prepared for the fourth Healthy Cities Symposium in Pècs (Hungary), Eindhoven: Municipal Public Health Services.

Gribling, A. (1990) *A Healthy School in a Healthy Community. The Environment Project in Eindhoven*, Paper prepared for the fifth Healthy Cities Symposium in Stockholm. Eindhoven: Municipal Public Health Services.

Harberden, P. van and Lafaille, R. (eds) (1979) *Zelfhulp, een nieuwe vorm van hulpverlening?* Vuga, 's-Gravenhage.

Kamp, J. van der (1985) *Informele Zorg. Uitgangspunten voor beleid inzake de informele zorg in het kader van het volksgezondheidsbeleid in Eindhoven*, Eindhoven: GGD Eindhoven.

Kamp, J. van der (1989) *Strengthening Health Involvement through Trends in Society*, Paper prepared for the fourth Healthy Cities Symposium in Pècs (Hungary), Eindhoven: Municipal Public Health Services.

Kamp, J. van der (1990a) *Action for Health: From Opponents to Partners*, Paper prepared for the fifth Healthy Cities Symposium in Stockholm, Eindhoven: The Netherlands Healthy Cities Network.

Kamp, J. van der (1990b) 'Managing Health Promotion as an Open Process', in A. Evers, W. Farrant and A. Trojan (eds) *Healthy Public Policy at the Local Level*, European Centre for Social Welfare and Policy Research, Frankfurt: Campus Verlag.

Kamp, J. van der and Cosijn, J. (1987) *Health Promotion. The Nota 2000 Applied to Setting the Course for Health Promotion and Health Education in Eindhoven*, Eindhoven: Municipal Public Health Services.

Kickbusch, I. and Hatch, S. (1983) 'A Reorientation of Health Care?', in I. Kickbusch and S. Hatch (eds) *Self-help and health in Europe*, Copenhagen: World Health Organization Regional Office for Europe.

Leeuw, E. de (1989) *The Sane Revolution. Health Promotion: Backgrounds, Scope, Prospects*, Assen/Maastricht: Van Gorcum.

Mayor's Survey (1984) *KidsPlace: Technical Report*, Washington.

WVC, Ministerie van Welzijn, Volksgezondheid en Cultuur (1986) *Nota 2000. Gezondheid als uitgangspunt*, Tweede Kamer, vergaderjaar 1985/1986, kamerstuk 19 500, nrs 1-2-3.

15

Barcelona

Jaume Costa

Genesis of the project

In June 1986 the Barcelona City Council agreed to take part in the World Health Organization (WHO) Healthy Cities Project. This official decision was the result of a lengthy process. Two of the city's public health agencies, the Municipal Health Institute (MHI) and the Barcelona Municipal Laboratory, had been in existence for almost one hundred years, and the two centres have been among Spain's most active and innovative agencies in the area of public health in recent years. Their quality during the Franco dictatorship, as with that of public administration as a whole, had been considerably diminished in comparison with other countries. In addition, the appearance of new medical technologies and the growth of the hospital sector had pushed public health issues to one side. The return to a democratic system permitted a renewal of the institutions of local government. In the City Health Department, a deep change started after the first democratic municipal elections in 1979. The Public Health Councillor set out the priorities for the city's public health policy (Clos 1987):

1 to introduce a health promotion perspective in the city political agenda
2 to encourage a cultural change in health-related attitudes and behaviours
3 to adapt health care services to population needs
4 to enable the organization of a future Catalan Health Service.

These priorities form part of a general framework for the improvement of management effectiveness, concern for the quality of services provided, and the promotion of citizen participation in health care issues. Thus, services in both public health and environmental protection have been integrated into a single organizational structure, activities have been arranged into programmes, indicators have been designed to monitor these programmes, and mechanisms for continuing professional education have been established.

A thoroughgoing renewal of personnel took place at the same time. The strict application of the Law on Incompatible Activities led to the resignation of a large number of city employees, and younger doctors occupied their places. Many of these new doctors have studied Master's level public health courses in the United States, Britain, France and Belgium, or have specialized in family and community medicine. These professionals returned to Spain with a public health concept much broader than the narrow microbiological focus on controlling transmittable diseases, and they proposed new approaches that combined disciplines as varied as epidemiology, statistics, health programme planning and health promotion.

It was within this context that the Public Health Councillor submitted to the City Council a proposal to join the WHO Healthy Cities Project. This coincided with Barcelona city health policy goals stated after the first democratic elections: It is clear that public health will be improved by decisions that are made outside the health sector (every decision that increases the educational level, the quality of life, the freedom and solidarity of the general public, will also improve health), and that is why health is, first of all, a political matter, and only secondarily a technical one. The contemporary view in Barcelona is that health should be not only an issue of experts but also an endeavour, through organizations and institutions, of each individual, on the one hand, and of society as a whole, on the other.

Elements of the Project

In Barcelona, the Healthy Cities Project has legitimized and reinforced the city health policies and enriched them with the ideas and experiences of other European cities. The elements of the project may be classified according to the priorities of the municipal health policy.

To introduce a health promotion perspective in the city political agenda

A Health Promotion Division was created in 1986 within the framework of the MHI. Although it took over some of the activities that had traditionally been carried out by the MHI – such as vaccinations and medical check-ups for schoolchildren – the Division has started many new programmes and has restructured traditional ones, in accord with the New Public Health philosophy.

Even more important, however, was the introduction of the health promotion perspective into other city departments. For example, a committee staffed by members from the various municipal departments has developed an intersectoral plan to combat drug-abuse; the Sports Department and the Health Department organized an international symposium on 'Health and

Sports for All'; the Youth Department has accepted the responsibility for youth-related aspects of the Healthy Cities Project.

Furthermore, formal and informal contacts have been established between the City Health Department, community groups and the business sector. For instance, the Advisory Council on Occupational Health, composed of trade union members, employers, experts and politicians; the agreement made with savings banks to facilitate low-interest loans to industry and individuals for improvements in their fuel-burning facilities; agreements with the gas company to provide financial incentives for replacing polluting installations with gas burning units.

This health promotion perspective in the city health policy has also manifested itself in crisis situations. The best example is the asthma outbreaks caused by soybean powder. Since 1981, the emergency rooms of Barcelona's hospitals had been facing brief episodes of an increasing number of asthma cases. After several epidemiological and immunological studies (Antó and Sunyer 1986), it was discovered that these episodes coincided with the unloading of ships carrying soybean powder. The Mayor ordered the cancellation of all soybean-related harbour activity, despite strong pressure from the business sector. Changes were made in the unloading methods of the soybean, the asthma episodes disappeared and the Mayor again authorized the soybean unloading.

To encourage a cultural change in health-related attitudes and behaviours

Spain has no tradition of organized efforts to enable changes in behaviours. The Healthy Cities Project has developed an innovating role in this area as advocate and promoter of a new cultural attitude towards health. This innovative role is evident in the occupational sector. The Occupational Health Centre has prepared several programmes to quit smoking, employee training programmes to control risks in the work-place, programmes to reduce the causes and effects of stress.

In both the private and public sectors these programmes are models of good practice, and they are spreading a new cultural attitude towards health promotion in the work-place.

However, the project has almost always played the role of advocate. For International Health Day (7 April 1988) thousands of postcards asking people not to smoke on this day were sent all over the city. This initiative was presented to the mass media the same day, and over the following days the postcards of those who had agreed not to smoke on 7 April began to arrive at the City Health Department. Each smoker who had returned a postcard was sent a pamphlet with suggestions on how to quit smoking. The success of this initiative encouraged the City Health Department Director to propose to the Ministry of Health, the Autonomous Government of Catalonia, the Barcelona Olympic Organizing Committee and WHO, an agreement for 'Smoke Free Olympic Games', and this has been signed.

The municipal administration has often encouraged, with subsidies and technical support, activities of community groups aimed at improving health. This is the case with the citizens' groups involved with the prevention of AIDS, which organize 'safe sex' workshops, publish and distribute information brochures, and are concerned with assisting those who have tested HIV-seropositive. Another example of promoting a cultural change in relation to health is the Health Fair (Healthy Cities Centre 1989). This Fair demonstrated the influence of the physical and social environment on human health, and offered to the participants a variety of tests so they can check their own health.

To adapt health care services to population needs

The adaptation of health services to population needs is being implemented through the creation of a health information system, the introduction of health promotion into primary care services, and the development of self-help and self-care activities.

One of the first concerns of the democratic Health Department was the creation of a health information system that would indicate the population's health problems and the effectiveness of the health services. Objective data such as mortality and morbidity levels, hospital discharge diagnoses, and information about air pollution, are combined with subjective information such as that gathered in the home health survey, with measures of perceived morbidity, the use of health care services, and citizen's opinions about their own health or the Seattle KidsPlace (Mayor's Survey 1984).

Since 1984, the Health Department has submitted an annual report, *Health in Barcelona*, to the City Council, which provides the above information and sets the priorities for the coming year. The publication and distribution of this report enables Barcelona's citizens to learn of situations that are often overlooked, such as health inequalities among the city's various districts.

The introduction of health promotion in primary care services began with an anti-smoking counselling campaign conducted by the general practitioners of a primary care centre. This will permit an appropriate evaluation to be made, and consideration of extending the programme to other health centres in the future, perhaps to include additional topics such as physical exercise, alcohol and nutrition.

Activities are also being developed as an attempt to design a health care model beyond the traditional prescriptive one. In one initiative a questionnaire was mailed to self-help groups and personal interviews were conducted; the data obtained were used to prepare a guide to Barcelona's self-help groups. This guide will be distributed to health care and social services professionals, and also to the public. It will also be a useful tool for improving co-operation between health service agencies and the self-help groups.

Regarding self-care, a telephone survey has been planned that will gather data on self-care practices, and this will be the basis for a future self-care programme.

To enable the organization of a future Catalan Health Service

The General Health Law, passed by the Spanish Parliament in 1986, gives to the municipalities only responsibilities over the environment. Therefore, Barcelona's health services should be integrated into the unified structure of the Catalan Health Service. In addition to the public health services, this includes two general hospitals, a psychiatric centre, a geriatric centre, six family planning centres and two primary care centres.

Since the beginning of the city's first democratic government, the administrators of these centres have succeeded in controlling costs and increasing productivity. These policies have generated conflicts among the personnel and complaints by doctors to the mass media. However, this has enabled the reduction of the municipal budget percentage allocated to health care services. At the same time this restructuring of the municipal services was taking place, a technical committee was preparing a map of both public and private health care facilities. This group recommended that the city of Barcelona be organized as a single geographical health area, and divided into ten health sectors coinciding with the city's ten districts. This will permit the participation of the city's representatives in the Administrative Council of the health area, and in the boards of the health sectors. The Autonomous Government of Catalonia, at the city's request, has accepted this recommendation and the two administrations have signed an agreement on it.

Future Project developments

The municipal organizational structure is developing a process of decentralization and interdepartmental co-ordination. These two broad policies will influence the Project's future development. Under the new arrangements each city district is an administrative and political division. A councillor presides over a district council that co-ordinates the municipal programmes of the district. A significant portion of the resources, staff and budget, formerly assigned to the city's central departments, has been transferred to the districts. This will make intersectoral co-ordination and public participation easier. Within the general framework for decentralization, some programmes that were formerly run by the central Health Department are now implemented by the districts. Even more important, however, are the new horizontal programmes planned in some districts that co-ordinate public health with social services, educational services, youth services and sports services ... and also with neighbourhood associations and voluntary groups.

The co-ordination between central departments is both political and administrative. A deputy mayor co-ordinates the councillors of the various municipal departments included in a macro-department. The Health Department is part of the Social Welfare macro-department, which also includes the Social Services and Youth Department, the Education Department and the Sports Department. This organizational structure has facilitated horizontal plans (children, senior citizens, volunteers) that are being considered by the community groups concerned with the plan's subject, and by the municipal administration.

Thus, decentralization and macro-departments are organizational changes that are consistent with the Healthy Cities Project philosophy. A good example of their impact has been of that on urban noise, which is a major problem. The Health Department produced sonic maps; financial aid is available to reduce noise sources and transmission. However, the effectiveness of these strategies upon the noise levels was only relative. At present, in several districts citizens have formed commissions with the district's councillor to discuss the noise problems. It is probable that the participation of these citizens will give this problem priority status and will promote compliance with the noise control regulations, which often meet with great resistance when there is no community support behind them.

Another example of the influence of these policies in health is the case of the 'Old City' district. This district is Barcelona's poorest, with the highest percentage of immigrant and elderly populations, prostitution, old buildings in poor conditions. Health statistics show that this is the district with the highest infant mortality rates and lowest life expectancy, as well as the highest death-rate due to external causes. Decentralization has enabled the development of specific programmes to deal with the characteristics of this district. A mixed company has been set up with private and municipal capital for urban regeneration projects, several old buildings will be restored and converted into cultural centres for the entire city, new housing will be built, and some in poor condition will be remodelled. Programmes are also being implemented for the most vulnerable groups: mothers and children, intravenous drug users. The district's residents have played a very active role, particularly in some areas – such as the identification of the mafioso, for example.

The desire to move towards the future and define health policy objectives has led to the creation of a technical commission which has written a city health objectives proposal. This Commission has used as its starting-point the thirty-eight European targets of 'Health for All'. Health objectives will imply co-ordinated activities with community groups and the various government agencies. These co-ordinated activities, as models of good practice, should achieve visible results in the short term, reducing health inequalities and giving priority to prevention.

But at the same time that these plans are being made, there is also the desire to remain receptive to the opportunities offered by the future so that Barcelona may become a healthier city. This is a challenge that must be accepted by citizens, administrators and politicians if we want to achieve 'Health for All' in Barcelona.

References and further reading

Antó, J.M. and Sunyer, J. (1986) 'Asthma Collaborative Group: A Point Source Asthma Outbreak', *Lancet* 1: 900–3.

Clos, J. (1987) 'Pròleg' in *Programes d'Actuació*, Ajuntament de Barcelona. Barcelona: Àrea de Sanital, Salut Pública i Medi Ambiert.

Costa, J. and Moncada, S. (1989) 'The Advisory Council on Occupational Health – Barcelona', *Health Promotion* 4: 137–40.

Diez, E. and Plasencia, A. (1988) 'Maternal and Infant Care Program in a Deprived Urban Area', Paper prepared for the third Healthy Cities Symposium on Inequalities and Health, Zagreb (Yugoslavia).

Healthy Cities Centre (1989) 'Spanish Health Fair Pulls the Crowds', newsletter *Healthy Cities*, February, Liverpool: Healthy Cities Centre, Department of Public Health, University of Liverpool.

Mayor's Survey (1984) *KidsPlace: Technical Report*, Washington.

Roca, F. and Villalbi, J.R. (1989) 'Self help groups and organizations in Barcelona', Paper prepared for the fourth Healthy Cities Symposium on Community Health Action, Pècs (Hungary).

Spagnolo, E., Villalbi, J.R. and Costa, J. (1988) 'On the Development of Health Indicators for Cities: The Barcelona Experience', Paper prepared for the International Conference Health in Towns, Vienna.

Sunyer, J., Ant, J.M., Rodrigo, M.J. and Morell, F. (Clinical and epidemiological committee) (1989) 'Case-Control Study of Seroimmunoglobulin E Antibody Reactive with Soybean in Epidemic Asthma', *Lancet* 1: 179–82.

Villalbi, J.R., Costa, J. and Oller, N. (1988) 'Community Initiatives against AIDS in Barcelona', *Health Promotion* 4: 225–30.

16

The Basque Country

Ricardo Garcia Herrera and
Genaro Astray Mochales

Analysis of the situation

Spain is a country which is divided into seventeen autonomous communities or regions, which have administrative responsibilities in many policy areas, such as education, health and agriculture. The Basque Autonomous Community in the north of Spain has a common border with France (Figure 16.1) and is divided administratively in three historic territories (Instituto Vasco de Estadistica 1988): Alava (12 per cent of the population), Guipzcoa (33 per cent) and Vizcaya (55 per cent). The total population is 2.1 million, in an area of 7,261 km^2 with a population density of 294.18 inhabitants/km^2. It is an industrialized region with fifteen cities of over 25,000 inhabitants, which are home to 61.2 per cent of the population. Most of these cities expanded at a time of industrial growth, generating an aggressive urban environment with environmental deterioration, unemployment, drug addiction problems, and many other social problems. Characteristic of the cities is the way in which industry is incorporated in the town's structure, provoking a deterioration in the environment and a negative population perception. As a result residents have begun to demand strong intervention measures to oppose this environmental deterioration. In addition a large number of the psychosocial risk factors, such as unemployment, are still present as a result of the economic crisis of the 1970s. Of all these cities, only the capitals of the Historical Territories have the necessary technical equipment to analyse the environmental and health conditions of their populations. Others need technical assistance to develop a programme such as the 'Healthy Cities'. For this reason the Basque Government, through the Basque Health Service (OSAKIDETZA), decided to start the programme, encouraging the participation of local councils and giving them all kinds of information support. At the same time it

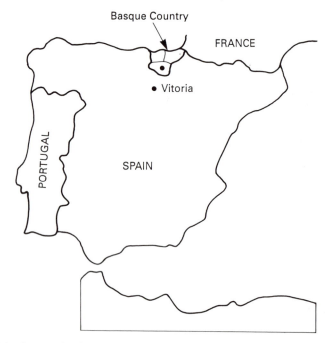

Figure 16.1   Geographic location and administrative division of the Basque Country.

provided important human, economic and technical resources to help the cities in the accomplishment of the programme. The Department of Health has also helped the local councils which have asked for assistance and has worked with them in a co-ordinated way to promote health in the cities.

In 1988 the Public Health Division of the Basque Department of Health and Consumer Affairs began a Public Health Programme covering the following areas: public drinking water, pesticides and chemical safety, radiology protection, beaches and swimming pools, sewage, food hygiene, zoonosis, slaughterers, occupational health, accidents, epidemic control and nutrition. The existence of these programmes helped the methodological development of the Healthy Cities programme and allowed the channelling of the different health problems existing in each city into a city diagnosis and health plan.

Strategy

Three lines of work have been established for the strategic development of the plan.

Promoting the Programme

Twenty local councils in the Basque Country have so far decided to take part in the programme. The Department of Health and Consumer Affairs has promoted the programme the following way:

1 A programme was drawn up adapted to the local situation of the Basque Country's local councils. It gave clear guidance as to the line of work to be assumed by the participants.
2 Once it had been approved, the programme was presented to the town's council, and studied by the local councillors. It was important to achieve a political consensus to facilitate the development and implementation of the programme. After the local council had approved the plan, the Mayor signed a collaboration agreement with the Basque Government's Health Department.
3 As next step the Department of Health undertook and financed the town's health risks analysis. Once these three steps had been embarked on the city could have access to subsidies and grants from the government to finance the public health problems prioritized in the town's study. As a fourth approach, larger towns, which had sufficient resources and services were able to control more directly their study and the programme. The main challenge for the Department of Health and Consumer Affairs was those towns of between 25,000 and 125,000 inhabitants which did not have sufficient structure to put the programme into operation.

Methodology

The Diagnostic Phase is based on each town's health risk analysis, including the environmental and social aspects. The main categories for description and analysis are as follows:

1 Environmental sectors
   • water
   • soil
   • air
   • plant life
   • energy
   • housing and city planning
   • socio-economic indicators
2 Analysis of negative health indicators
   • mortality rate
   • morbidity rate
3 Analysis of subjective or soft indicators – 'Perception of the City' – which is an attempt to determine the degree of acceptance residents have of their city
   • general perception of the city

- integration in the city
- perception of the town council's management of the city
- public space in the city
- social pessimism

4 Immediate surroundings, which defines the individuals' interactions with their immediate surroundings
- home
- family
- personal relationships
- work
- personality

5 Risk factor related behaviour, which refers to lifestyles considered as damaging for health
- drugs
- alcohol
- other drugs
- tobacco
- food
- health perception

6 Leisure and free time, which refers to the amount of free time available and how it is used
- active leisure time
- passive leisure time
- intellectual leisure time
- social leisure time

7 Needs, which tries to define the priorities for intervention expressed by the people interviewed
- environmental
- town planning
- public spaces
- cultural and social.

With these health indicators, objective and subjective factors were confirmed to obtain a joint vision of the state of the community and an appropriate plan for its health policies.

The health plan

Once the problems are identified, they are grouped into intervention strategies:

1 *Participative*: includes the different aspects of local life, as well as the different institutions acting in a particular area.
2 *Dynamic*: information strategies to enable responses to be made to changing events.
3 *Follow-up*: evaluation through objectives and indicators. As the local council is responsible for the implementation of the programme, the De-

partment of Health and Consumer Affairs will participate only if the council accepts the guidelines of the programme.

Training of the city health councillors

The regional government wanted local council representatives to be involved in the design of the plan, but before they could, it was found to be necessary for them to receive basic training in health planning and health promotion. With this idea in mind, in 1989 a continuous training workshop was set up for local politicians, consisting of more than one hundred hours of classes and fifteen conference sessions. This course enabled the local councillors responsible for health and the technicians of the Basque Health Service, to know each other and to work together, in the Healthy Cities programme.

After two years the programme has rapidly expanded, and now more than 65 per cent of the Basque population is included. In addition to that, risk analyses are available at municipal level allowing the detected problems to be given an order of priority.

Progress so far

Two different concepts of an ideal clean and healthy city emerged from our surveys. One was based on the opinions of the residents of the eight largest Basque towns, except Vitoria, and the other, more practical, being based on surveys undertaken in Vitoria-Gasteiz. Significant differences in mortality and morbidity rates in the highly industrialized areas of Vizcaya were identified and at the present time this is the main work priority.

What do residents consider a Healthy City?

When the project was started, one of the key questions was what do residents consider to be a Healthy City? A survey (Gobierno Vasco 1990) was carried out on residents of the eight largest Basque cities (2,188 questionnaires with a margin of error of 2.5 per cent and a confidence level of 95.5 per cent). The survey showed what people mostly considered to be an ideal healthy city (Figure 16.2):

1 An area completely free of pollution, with special emphasis on water, air and noise (88 per cent of the survey).
2 The existence of public areas for leisure-time activities as well as adequate medical services (50 per cent of the survey).
3 The improvement of the public transport network, working conditions, and citizens' information (30 per cent of the survey).
4 The desire that the residents' opinions be taken into consideration (30 per cent of the survey).

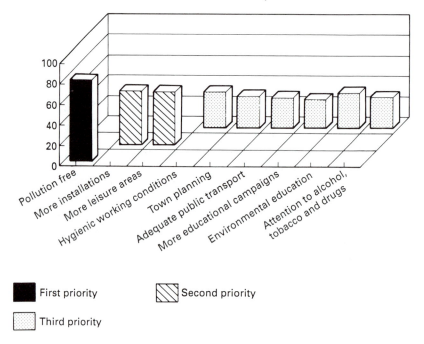

First priority   Second priority

Third priority

Figure 16.2   Priorities in a healthy city as seen by residents of eight Basque cities.

This variety of replies is a consequence of the city's objective realities, as we commented above, and no significant differences between the cities were found. On the other hand, differences do appear when we take age into consideration:

1 The youngest people surveyed (12–25 year olds) gave more importance to the existence of leisure and sports facilities (55 per cent).
2 Those over 65 gave special importance to an adequate health care system (55 per cent). The other priorities appeared in second place.

These differences in the two extreme age groups surveyed are logical and represent different expectations based on people's personal situation. On the other hand the perception of an ideal city is practically the same in all of the cities surveyed, keeping in touch with the reality of the Basque cities.

The example of Vitoria

The Vitoria health survey analysed the physical and social situation of the city, capital of the Autonomous Community with a population of 200,000. It identified intervention priorities for the following two years in a variety of fields. In order to implement these priorities an agreement was signed between the local council and the Department of Health and Consumer Affairs on 'Healthy Cities'. This document was divided into three parts.

The first part established the programmatic lines of the agreement, centred basically on the five action areas of the Ottawa Conference (WHO *et al.* 1986).

The second part set up a 'follow-up' commission, to monitor the programme's development, and provide the necessary information, to evaluate its progress. The commission has been formed from:

1 A President, the Mayor of Vitoria-Gasteiz.
2 Three Councillors responsible for the areas involved.
3 Two representatives from the Department of Health and Consumer Affairs.
4 Two representatives of neighbourhood committees and associations appointed by the Vitoria-Gasteiz town council.

In 1989 the Vitoria-Gasteiz local council agreed to set up a new Public Health Service, dedicated to:

1 Develop environmental protection plans encouraging the formation of local groups.
2 Promote healthy habits amongst the population.
3 Promote collaboration between the different departments in the city council in order to achieve a 'healthier city'.

On the other hand, the Department of Health and Consumer Affairs agreed to co-ordinate the Healthy Cities Programme by:

1 Giving technical and informative advice on the activities to be carried out by the local Health Department.
2 Carrying out Vitoria's health risk analysis.
3 Supporting demands of the city to obtain funds from other Departments of the Basque Government involved in the Healthy Cities Programme.

Finally, in the third part of the agreement, an intervention plan was proposed for 1989 based on the problems detected in the environmental health survey. It proposed a series of specific actions in all the analysed sectors. The local council agreed to commission a public health expert and a technician to work on the programme. They were to be located at the local Institute of Health and Consumer Affairs. Examples of the environmental agreements reached are as follows:

1 drinking water
2 liquid waste
3 solid waste
4 noise
5 fauna and food hygiene
6 atmospheric pollution
7 other areas
8 social area.

These eight examples will now be discussed in turn.

Drinking water

Problems were detected in the reservoirs, where water is collected to supply Vitoria. These were not adequately protected and increased eutrophization and chemical pollution was found. Part of the water was not filtered, and high levels of lambliasis were recorded in the infant population. Once the problem was known it was given priority and action was taken by the organizations responsible in this area. A multisectoral commission was created to analyse the problem.

Liquid waste

Sixteen companies working in the area were found to be disposing of chemical wastes with high heavy metals content. Once the situation was known the responsibilities of the organizations participating in the agreement were discussed. The town council decided to control the dumping of wastes.

Solid waste

The following problems were detected in the city's legal dump site:

1 Run-off water circulates in the open air and discharges directly into a small river running nearby.
2 The dump-site is not isolated and no check of the incoming wastes is carried out.

On the other side around the city many illegal waste sites were detected with no control at all of the source and content of the wastes. An intervention programme was designed. After two years of work the problems have been solved.

Noise

The Local Council of Vitoria-Gasteiz approved an Order to control the acoustic level in the city. A study of the noise problem in the city was carried out and a city acoustic map was drawn. The town council has begun a campaign to make the public aware of this problem.

Fauna and food hygiene

The inspection and control of food in Vitoria-Gasteiz was considered adequate; nevertheless, the local council collaborates in any way necessary with the territory's Health Department, specifically in salmonellosis and other food-related programmes (retail trade, transport, microbiological meat control, and animal health).

Atmospheric pollution

In 1989 the Vitoria-Gasteiz local council increased the number of pollutants monitored; for the first time NOx, CO and hydrocarbons were included. An atmospheric clean-up plan for the local area was also studied. Its viability will be decided next year. The relocation of the company FUNDIX S.A. (the only company situated within the town area) was decided as a consequence of an agreement between the local council and the company. It left its location on 31 December 1989.

Other areas

Any special action necessary will be carried out in programmes already underway such as drug addiction (alcoholism, smoking, etc.). Information programmes were designed to improve the population's behaviour towards cleaner surroundings, pollution, healthy habits, lifestyles, etc.

Social area

The Department of Health of the Basque Government and the Public Health Service of Vitoria-Gasteiz are going to carry out a study in the local area of how to encourage the necessary participation of the population in the Healthy City programme.

Population perception

According to its residents, not only does Vitoria-Gasteiz have a need to improve its environment through such things as greening, but also people feel a great need for improving its social aspects. Vitoria is a new city, which had a high population growth in the 1970s (its second reindustrialization). Its surroundings have been unaltered but this contributes to other problems, such as the absence of real social networks in the city, which could help in difficult family situations or personal problems.

This problem can be studied only from the point of view of social science and it is so important that we cannot seriously approach the planning or the development of local health policies, without taking into consideration, local psychosocial realities. For this reason, it is necessary to have access to indicators which can condense all the information available. We also need some reference levels and points of comparison between cities. The situation can be briefly explained for Vitoria-Gasteiz, using only two indicators, 'the general indicator of city perception' and the 'citizens' demands' indicator (at the present time we are working with twenty-four subjective indicators), which we think sum up the overall reality.

These indicators stem from the analysis of opinion polls specifically designed

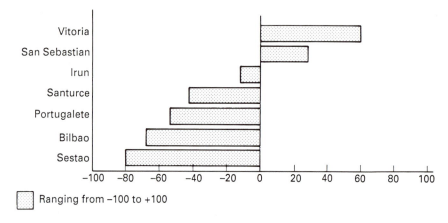

Figure 16.3 The general perception index in eight Basque cities.

to work with a multivariant analysis and subsequently to draw up complex indices. Therefore we have indicators which are peculiar and unique to each local council, and others which are general indicators. The city perception's general indicator refers to the real perception people have of their city, that is, it is a measure of the city's objective environmental situation (clean city, polluted, noisy, overpopulated, built-up, installations, etc.). This indicator makes each individual take a clearly negative or positive attitude towards their city, giving a global value from which it is difficult to extract all its components. The general perception index is a value between -100 (all of the people interviewed have a negative image of the city) to $+100$ (all of the people interviewed have a positive image of the city). The average of the eight cities studied was 31.7. This shows a generally negative perception, and makes us think about the environmental situation of the cities (Figure 16.3). The variance analysis indicates that there are significant differences between the perceptions of the different cities analysed. In Vitoria-Gasteiz, the reading was 59.8, showing a city with the best perception of its surroundings, followed by San Sebastian, with an index of 27.0, whilst the rest of the cities have negative values, Bilbao (-68.6) and Sestao (-79.9).

The factors which weigh most in this negative impression are noise (-46.2) and atmospheric pollution (-37.2). If the scores given to the general index and the pollution level are analysed, there is a high correlation between them, hence the 'Pearson r' is 0.9874, which indicates that 97.7 per cent ($r2$) of the general index can be explained by the perception or non-perception of pollution and vice-versa. (The Pearson r is a statistical measure of the strength of correlation between two factors.)

In any case, if the index is analysed by its different components in Vitoria they are all positive (healthy, clean, little pollution, somewhat noisy, not overpopulated, good town planning and adequate facilities) (Figure 16.4), obtaining the lowest values for noise $(+9.1)$. The industrial cities give nega-

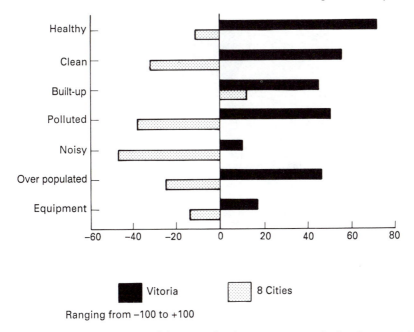

Figure 16.4 The components of the general index, in Vitoria and other Basque cities.

tive results in all these factors. The 'citizens' demands' indicator attempts to explain the needs felt by the population. Five factors are considered, pollution – including air, water and noise pollution – road and traffic improvements, improvements in education, improvement in free time facilities, and drug control. Vitoria-Gasteiz (Figure 16.5) 36.2 per cent of the replies were for a reinforcement of measures to reduce general pollution. If we consider the different types of pollution, we find that 15 per cent wanted atmospheric pollution to be reduced (in industrial areas this was over 30 per cent), 7.7 per cent noise pollution and 7.4 per cent water pollution. Education, with 23.5 per cent was the second factor amongst the population demands of Vitoria. Alcohol, tobacco and drugs control came in third place. In fourth place were improvements in the traffic situation (17.5 per cent); 9.4 per cent indicated the need to improve the public transport system. The improvement of facilities was in last place (10.4 per cent), unlike other cities in the Basque Country, where it was first.

From a closer examination of the surveys, it is worth noting that complaints about pollution in Vitoria are ten points below the average, and in the case of free-time facilities, almost seven points below. The opposite is the case in the need for an improvement in education and drug control.

Thus we are faced with two different types of cities: those which have not solved the problems considered by the population as important or primary (showing a negative perception index) and those with a positive perception,

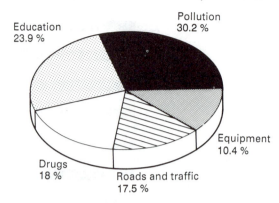

Figure 16.5 Indicator of population demands in Vitoria.

where the priority demands of the population may be considered as secondary: access to information, the need for children's education, problems with drug, tobacco or alcohol consumption, or the development of areas for leisure-time activities.

The development of these indicators has changed the situation in Vitoria. All the problems discussed in the agreement have been or are going to be solved soon and in a very efficient way. There has also been an important change in the priorities of the city's health department. Before, they had been basically centred around the city's hygiene problems. Now priority is given to an improvement in lifestyle (alcohol, tobacco, etc.), and other problems which may influence the life-quality of its citizens. Two years after the project began, we are now convinced that it has had a positive effect, not only in Vitoria-Gasteiz, which is a well-planned city and an example of good local administration in our country but also for the rest of the local councils taking part in the programme.

References

Gobierno Uasco (1990) *Las ciudades saludables en Euskadi.* Serie Documentos Tecnicos de Salud Publica, numero 7, Vitoria.
Instituto Vasco de Estadistica – EUSTAT (1988) *Anuario Estadistico Vasco*, pp 35–120, Vitoria: EUSTAT.
WHO (World Health Organisation), Health and Welfare Canada, Canadian Public Health Association (1986) *Ottawa Charter for Health Promotion*, Copenhagen: WHO.

17

Valencia

*Carlos Alvarez-Dardet and
Concha Colomer*

Background

The Valencian Community is one of the seventeen Spanish autonomous regions. It is located on the Mediterranean coast and has around 4 million inhabitants, roughly one-tenth of the Spanish population; 72 per cent of the people live in urban areas. A wide range of economic and population trends can be observed within the Valencian community's cities. The economic crisis of some industries has led to the decline of several cities whereas other cities have flourished precisely because of the nature of their local economy. The cities on the coast are generally richer and more populated as a result of tourism and agricultural activities.

Valencia is one of the regions where the Spanish National Health Service has a decentralized budget. Although the larger cities such as Valencia or Alicante have municipal public health services, the public health functions are in the most part covered by services delivered through the Regional Health System. Since the end of Franco's dictatorship and especially under the years of Socialist government in Spain there has been a renaissance of public health with the creation of many new services and since 1984 the establishment of four new Schools of Public Health in Granada, Pamplona, Valencia and Madrid.

Starting-point

By means of the personal contacts maintained with two participating cities in the WHO-Network (Liverpool and Barcelona) a group of academics started to develop the Healthy Cities ideas in our region in the spring of 1987 from two institutions: the Department of Community Health of the University of Alicante and the Valencian School of Public Health in Valencia (IVESP).

Spreading the Healthy Cities idea and concepts among public health workers, politicians and the community at large was considered as an important priority. The fact that all the printed pertinent material was produced in English seriously hindered attaining this objective. The sometimes tedious translation into Spanish of two books on Healthy Cities (Ashton 1987) and the New Public Health (Ashton and Seymour 1990) as well as the production of pamphlets, teaching material and a newsletter have been important parts of our work during the past two years.

Inside the Valencian Community, support was obtained from the local governments, especially those of Alicante, Elche and Alcoy and the Valencian Federation of Provinces and Municipalities. The most important support was obtained from the Generalitat Valenciana (the Regional Government) that by founding the co-ordinating office and giving political support contributed significantly to determining the current political visibility of the Valencian network of Healthy Cities.

Outside the Spanish borders we have found advisership, collaboration and in some way a source of legitimation by actively participating in informal networks related to Healthy Cities particularly in academic circles.

Our experience has shown that although the official relationship with international bureaucracies may be important, they are neither sufficient nor necessary to be able to act locally in the Healthy Cities style.

The Valencian network of Healthy Cities, which now has thirty-four member cities, has two co-ordinating offices in the cities of Valencia and Alicante staffed by two full-time professionals trained in public health and two part-time honorary senior consultants. It has organized three annual meetings and is involved in a wide variety of activities with the Town Halls of the participating cities, the public health professionals, the universities of the region, the Health Services and community groups.

In order to offer an overall view of the process developed in the Valencian Community, which has progressed, at times failed and fluctuated throughout these years, the seven tasks for the participating cities stated in the early stages of the project will be used as a check-list in the following manner:

High-level intersectoral groups

Although the creation and maintenance of intersectoral groups at a top political level occurs in a formal way in many of the participating cities, the degree of commitment and its usefulness varies widely from one city to another and depends largely on the beliefs of the political leader of the city in the Healthy Cities ideas. Up until now we feel that although many interesting things are occurring in a group of cities, these developments are relatively independent of the efforts made by the co-ordinating group and are more strongly connected with the political situation of the city and with different leadership roles.

An interesting experience of the potential effect of intersectoral committees which has been successful in developing ecological strategies has taken place in Silla, a town near Valencia, where a high level of environmental pollution led to the radical management of the problem of contaminating factories.

Technical intersectoral groups

The lack of public health professionals appointed at the city level greatly limited the development of a group of professionals who could support the activities in the cities from a technical point of view.

Some measures have been developed to overcome this limitation. The Regional Government of Valencia and some municipalities have provided funds or developed links with academic institutions such as the Schools of Medicine and Nursing or the School of Public Health and also with private public health consultants to meet their needs.

Nevertheless there is an evident and clear need for a major involvement of the Regional Health Services (Servei Valencia de Salut) and its public health services in this task of accommodating creatively the local needs and the regional budget to each other.

Community diagnosis

Several municipal governments (Elche, Alicante, Elda, Petrel), the provincial government of Valencia (Diputación) and the Regional Government (Generalitat) have provided funds to develop community diagnoses at the city level.

Some of them have already been completed and published and others are still in the stages of fieldwork or planning. The universities of the region and the School of Public Health (IVESP) have provided the technical resources for this task. In 1989 the IVESP organized a workshop to discuss the common bases of the community diagnosis in the region, this working party developed a check-list of ten points as recommendations for the community diagnoses in the Valencian network of Healthy Cities:

1 The community diagnosis should be orientated and based on health and not on diseases, as a part of a continuous process.
2 There is a remarkable lack of municipal databases which should be created as soon as possible.
3 If the diagnosis is made by an intersectoral group it permits a better understanding of the city status.
4 The inequalities in health should be evidenced by the community diag-

nosis which should make comparisons between the different groups in the city as well as compare status in the city with that in other cities.

5 The community diagnosis can be seen as a tool for community participation, this means recognizing that the gathered information belongs to the community. Accordingly, transmitting the information to the community became the most important objective.

6 The report should be understood by people without special training in medicine or in the health sciences. It should be a short, clear and concise report and not a long list of problems.

7 The ultimate goal of this kind of report is to develop a debate about health in the city. To attain it the report should be based on information which is of interest both to politicians and the community.

8 The mass media should participate in spreading the information. The additional use of marketing techniques permits a better diffusion of the reports.

9 A community debate about the conclusions following the diagnosis should be actively encouraged in those community groups with no political affiliation (including children and teenagers).

10 The feasibility of the priorities established in the community diagnosis should be guaranteed by actively negotiating with the different groups which represent conflicting interests in the city.

Links between the city and the educational institutions

The creation of links with educational institutions has been easily developed because of the importance that academics had in introducing the Healthy Cities strategy in our region. A wide range of activities has been developed in the areas of teaching, research and in visibly portraying Healthy Cities among public health professionals.

Seminars on Healthy Cities are considered as a part of undergraduate studies in the school of social workers, in the Schools of Nursing, as an important part of the Master's degree programme in the School of Public Health and in the Doctorate programme of the Department of Community Health of the University of Alicante. Five international courses have been organized in the School of Public Health along with a yearly course in the Menorca's Summer School of Public Health.

Several research projects, some of them as a fruit of international co-operation, are in progress on indicators and nutrition, and take their place along with the analysis of a large Healthy Cities household survey with more than 2,000 interviews.

To disseminate the Healthy Cities approach among public health professionals the annual meeting is extensively publicized and has become an annual meeting point in the region, as the 1988 meeting with more than 100 submitted papers shows. With the same idea and as a response to our initiative, the journal of the Spanish Public Health Association (*Gaceta Sanitaria*) has now created a Healthy Cities Section.

Models of good practice

The projects or experiences which are within the scope of Healthy Cities in the Valencian Community largely reflect the underlying political situation and the changes produced in the practice of public health in recent years.

The almost complete lack of community organizations in Spain, compared with other countries whose democratic tradition dates further back, has been pointed out by many political analysts in our country and can probably be attributed to the effect of the Franco-prolonged dictatorship on civil society. Another important fact which affects the development of models of good practice in Spain is the current situation of the Public Health Services with vertical programmes and until very recently strongly orientated towards infectious disease prevention, on the other hand the organization of the Public Health Services by including them in the health care system in 1988 has produced many new opportunities as well as problems.

In spite of this situation and especially during 1989 many previously untapped experiences became visible as a result of the creation of the Healthy Cities arena for discussion.

Some of these have been initiated by local government, such as the process of discussion and negotiation of Benidorm Town Hall with the owners of the tobacconist shops to use the taxes obtained by these shops in anti-tobacco campaigns. Others were initiated elsewhere such as the Godella elderly women experience which is a pioneer physical fitness programme in our region developed by a primary health care midwife. But the kind of projects which appear in the Healthy Cities literature and which are truly horizontal, belonging to the community, are still missing to a great extent in our community.

Health debate

Obviously the mass media should be used as the means to generate a debate about any topic. In these three years we have learned a lot by working with communication professionals mainly about the greatly different results obtained if one tries to 'use' the mass media or if one tries to involve the mass media in the process.

Several journalists from the press, television and radio are now connected with the co-ordinating Health Cities centres within a 'Healthy Cities Association' which has recently been created and meets every month. As a result of this involvement several projects are under way and a weekly Healthy Cities radio programme is broadcast throughout a regional radio station.

The local newspapers have also played an important role publishing news from the co-ordinating offices as well as the results of the community diagnosis. The debate on Healthy Cities has even reached the regional parliament, where an official session has been devoted to the progress of Healthy Cities in the Valencian Community reflecting the wide interest the debate has aroused among the people of the region.

The city of the Valencian network which has advanced the most in its health debate is probably the city of Elche. It has produced a set of twelve priorities based on the thirty-eight WHO targets and its own community diagnosis. A group of professionals, local politicians, MPs, representatives from health and social services, from women's and consumer's associations and several journalists produced the following statement as a proposal for public debate (Silvestre *et al.* 1990):

By understanding health as a state of physical, psychological and social well-being and not merely as the absence of disease, we reaffirm the urgent need to eliminate those remaining situations in the city considered as prerequisites for health by the WHO such as the elimination of deprivation and slum housing.

At the same time, we consider health to be a resource for the quality of everyday life and from this perspective propose that Elche should begin a debate on the health of the city taking the following priorities into account:

1 To stimulate and facilitate healthy lifestyles.
2 To reduce health inequalities generated by socio-economic status, age and sex by developing positive interventions which favour equity.
3 To encourage the social structures of mutual, self-help and voluntary help groups.
4 To carry out specific actions against drug abuse in all the age groups and for all types of drugs.
5 To encourage physical exercise in all the groups within the population.
6 To improve the quality of housing and ensure accessibility to proper houses at affordable prices.
7 To reduce the cost in health produced by motor traffic.
8 To improve working conditions and occupational health.
9 To develop health promotion programmes in the school population.
10 To ensure that environmental and health needs are taken into account when decisions in the city and strategic planning are made.
11 To favour primary health care, social services and community health as the axes of the care system.
12 To stimulate the community to participate in the 'Healthy Cities Project'.

Mutual support

The annual meeting together with administrative meetings and the *Ciudades Sanas* newsletter are the ways by which experiences are communicated and links of collaboration among cities are developed.

Our group has been extensively involved in propagating the Healthy Cities ideas and concepts to the Spanish-speaking countries. Consequently as a result of an agreement reached among the publishers of the *Healthy Cities Newsletter* in Liverpool, the IVESP and PAHO (Pan American Health Organization) office in Washington. The *Ciudades Sanas* newsletter is now being distributed throughout Central and South America. The Spanish edition of this newsletter publishes the same material as the English one but adds information of special interest for Spanish-speaking countries (see Plate 17.1).

Concluding remarks

A movement which was similar to some extent to the current Healthy Cities Project was developed at the end of the nineteenth century in the city of Alicante under the leadership of José Gadea, who besides being an architect and a medical doctor held the office of Mayor of Alicante for several years. His writings (Gadea 1894, 1913) have been rescued and extensively studied by Professor Rosa Ballester (1991), who has also analysed the reasons why such a historical antecedent failed when it was put into practice. None of the revolutionary ideas of Gadea connected effectively with the social and political trends of his time. Gadea's lack of political power prevented him from imposing his ideas using a paternalistic approach and the result, at the turn of the century, was a city quite different from Gadea's Utopia.

Looking at the past we can identify some issues related to policy strategies and community participation which can affect the success of our efforts to change the environment of the cities and the lifestyles of the population. These issues are summarized as follows:

1 To develop a process of negotiation to produce an explicit political strategy on Healthy Cities at the local level.
2 To define the role of the health services in the Healthy Cities movement.
3 To go further with the idea of 'Thinking globally and acting locally', which is the 1990 slogan of WHO, and after achieving this go on to 'Think locally and act globally', by looking for new ways of international co-operation, in a more flexible and effective way.

References

Ashton, J. (1987) *La Promoción de la Salud: Un nuevo concepto para la nueva sanidad*, Generalitat Valenciana. Monografies Sanitaries Serie D. no. 1.
Ashton, J. and Seymour, H. (1988) *The New Public Health*, Milton Keynes: Open University Press.

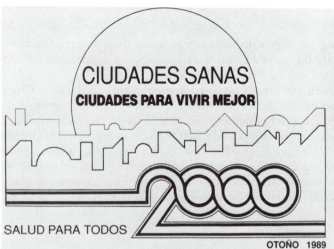

CIUDADES SANAS
CIUDADES PARA VIVIR MEJOR

SALUD PARA TODOS

2000

OTOÑO 1989

Publicación editada por el Centro de Ciudades Sanas de intercambio de información

Versión en español editada por el **Instituto Valenciano de Estudios en Salud Pública (IVESP)**. España. En colaboración con la asesoría regional de educación para la Salud de la **Oficina Sanitaria Panamericana (OPS) Organización Mundial de la Salud (OMS)** Washington. EEUU.
(Traducción M.ª Isabel Sans. Escuela de Enfermería, Universidad de Alicante España)

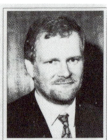

Carta del Editor

Muchas gracias a todos los que han contribuido en este ejemplar.

Siguiendo con lo que mencionábamos en el último, en el que enfatizábamos el contingente de planes introducidos para "limpiar la escena" de droga en un intento de evitar la propagación del SIDA, hacemos mención aquí a dos nuevos programas iniciados en Nueva Gales del Sur. Se trata de más canjes de agujas y jeringas a nivel farmacéutico. El número de las mismas distribuidas a usuarios de drogas por vía intravenosa, el año pasado, vino a oscilar entre el millón y el millón y medio. En 1990, el objetivo es llegar a los 9 millones.

Sin movernos de Australia, Ciudades Sanas informa del creciente éxito de la red australiana. El coordinador de Proyecto Nacional, Lewis Kaplan, hace una serie de consideraciones muy valiosas en su resumen de la situación allí. Con respecto a un proyecto específico, el de "Localidades Sanas" de Victoria, él aplaude el incentivo económico propuesto para aquellas poblaciones o localidades que deseen adherirse al compromiso de finalidades y objetivos del Proyecto Nacional, de lo que –en su opinión– adolece Ciudades Sanas. Las corporaciones locales pueden parecer, en ocasiones, un tanto remisas a la hora de adoptar nuevas ideas o nuevos enfoques en cuanto a promociones de salud se refiere, y es porque tienden a enfocarlos en términos de meros proyectos que exigen un esfuerzo económico, más que en nuevas orientaciones que precisan simplemente de unos recursos. (El informe completo del Sr. Kaplan, se puede leer en las páginas interiores).

Como consecuencia de las conversaciones mantenidas con colegas de todo el mundo, me doy cuenta de que existe un gran número de planteamientos de los que vale la pena informarse. Si, de alguna manera, alguien de Vds. está desarrollando o se le ocurre algún proyecto que pueda suponer una contribución a Ciudades Sanas, le ruego me envíe unas líneas. Permítanme que vuelva a incidir en un par de cuestiones que considero importantes: una es la importancia de compartir sus experiencias con las de otras gentes al objeto de que todos aprendamos de todos, y la segunda cuestión es simplemente recordarles que Ciudades Sanas es su periódico. Mantengamos una comunicación fluida. Muchas gracias.

Howard Seymour

Editor

La dirección es:
Editor de Ciudades Sanas.
Normanton Grange,
Langham Avenue, Aigburth.
Liverpool, L17

La Tragedia de Hillsborough

por el Dr. John Ashton

En una Ciudad Sana los padres podrán dejar que sus hijos asistan a un partido de fútbol sabiendo que volverán a casa sanos y salvos. Ese no fue el caso de Sheffield, el 15 de abril cuando 95 personas, muchas de ellas jóvenes e incluso un niño de 10 años, resultaron muertas en el peor desastre deportivo que se haya visto jamás en Gran Bretaña.

Las repercusiones inmediatas no se hicieron esperar: la especulación con las entradas, el mal estado del campo –falto de las más elementales normas de seguri-dad–, la necesidad de respuesta urgente desde un punto de vista político está siendo examinada muy de cerca, pero lo que nos llama la atención y subyace, es el modo en que la sociedad se pronuncia con respecto a los jóvenes en particular y más específicamente a los seguidores del fútbol. Parece como si en los últimos años constituyeran una subespecie humana, a la que hay que controlar y contener.

(Continúa en la página 2)

¡ULTIMA HORA!

La Paz (Bolivia) Pionera del Movimiento Ciudades Sanas en Latinoamérica

(más información en pág. 9)

Figure 17.1   The front cover of a recent Spanish version of the Healthy Cities Newsletter.

Ashton, J. and Seymour, H. (1990) *La Nueva Salud Pública*, Barcelona: Masson.

Ballester, R. (1991) 'Los aspectos sanitarios en el movimiento de desarrollo y reforma de las ciudades Europeas (1870–1925)'. I Colloquio interdepartamental Ciudad e Ideologia. Valencia Conselleria de Industria e Instituto Juan Gil Albert.

Colomer, C. and Costa, J. (1989) 'El programa ciudades Saludables en España', *Revisiones en Salud Pública* 1: 159–74.

Costa, J. and Alvarez-Dardet, C. (1989) 'Ciudades Saludables: Un movimiento para la Nueva Salud Pública', *Gaceta Sanitaria* 3(12): 407.

Gadea y Pro J. (1894) 'Informe resumen de las memorias presentadas por las Juntas Municipales'. Alicante, Establecimiento Tipográfico 'El Graduador'.

Gadea y Pro J. (1913) 'Reglamento para la Higiene y Salubridad de la ciudad de Alicante'. Alicante Imprime Such y Serra.

IVESP (1989) *Recomendaciones para la realización y difusión de diagnósticos de salud*, Red Ciudades Sanas de la Comunidad Valenciana.

Silvestre, A., Peiro, R., Tuells, J. *et al.* (1990) 'Utilización de un método de consenso para la determinación de las necesidades de Salud en Elche', *Gaceta Sanitaria* 4(18): 121–3.

Tsouros, A. (1991) *El Proyecto Ciudades Sanas de la O.M.S.*, Valencia: Instituto Valenciano de Estudios en Salud Pública.

18

Zagreb

*S. Sogoric, S. Ferint, S. Lang
and M. Dobranovi*

Introduction

The Zagreb, Yugoslavia, concept of the Healthy City represents a special model within the European project. The activities of most of the cities involved in the Project are often limited by territory (they are taking place only in some cities' districts), by the population (orientated only towards some of the population groups) and by the problems they solve (solving only one or more public health problems). The Zagreb model, however, is unlimited, and is open to a flow of ideas, people and activities. The project is participatory, voluntary, orientated towards the city's residents, belongs to everyone and has no experts who are working exclusively on this project.

There are, of course, experts working in the project but through their institutions and from the positions they have held in them from before the Healthy City Project started. The activities of the projects are orientated towards a wide spectrum of public health problems chosen by the Zagreb citizens themselves.

In 1987 Zagreb joined the Healthy Cities movement but the activities which led to this involvement had begun many years before. Through the work of Professor Andrija Stampar, the School of Public Health and other institutions such as the Institute for Public Health and Health Centres for primary health care, Zagreb has for a long time been a source of public health tradition and experience. When we started the project in Zagreb we had people with a long history of voluntary activities and a strong demand for change in the field of health. There have been a lot of obstacles to our project since the beginning such as foreign debt and economic and political crises which have made the challenge even greater.

Although the WHO Global Targets are central to the Zagreb approach, the question as to the manner in which the project addresses them remains open. The main issues in the Zagreb Healthy Cities Project are as follows:

1 Our citizens are our biggest resource – their knowledge, experience, energy and variety is what must be drawn upon. The question is how to find them, how to raise their interest for participation in the project and how to involve them in the project?
2 Co-operation and co-ordination are the prerequisites for success. How can we unify all the efforts in the community and involve people in a Zagreb network of people and groups working for health?
3 Health is a resource for everyday living. Healthy living is a prerequisite for prosperity. How do we make healthier lifestyles easily accessible to all people?

Project structure: project network

Inside the project we have established two methods of putting together community forces orientated towards health promotion in the city:

1 Territorial health promotion boards, which are located in the fourteen Zagreb communities.
2 Thematic groups, which were established in order to cover the leading public health problems in the city and vulnerable groups in the town population.

The 'umbrella' covering all Healthy City activities is the Health Assembly established on 7 April 1989, on World Health Day. The Health Assembly convenes once a year, bringing together the health promoting forces (in the broadest sense) of the city. At the first Health Assembly we discussed health promotion activities and future plans for every commune of the city of Zagreb.

The main topic of the Second Health Assembly was the human environment. For this occasion the Healthy Cities Project groups organized a poster exhibition which showed the leading activities for the improvement of the quality of environment which took place during 1989/90. The introductory reports will present the problems and directions for future activities with the same goal.

During the year, the Health Assembly runs the project activities through its working boards: a presidential board, executive board and project co-ordinating board. Territorial health promoting boards were formed in all fourteen communes of Zagreb, at the initial meeting held in February 1989. The members of the boards are representatives of the formal public and political organizations, factories, schools, cultural centres and health centres as well as the representatives from the informal groups and organizations.

In the first phase of their activities the boards had the task of answering the following questions presenting the situation in their commune:

1 Which are the health promoting forces in their commune and how do they mobilize them?
2 Which are the existing health promoting programmes (models of good practice)?
3 Which are the leading public health problems in their commune?

In the second phase the boards have agreed upon the directions for their further activities and have designed strategies for their implementation. In the setting up of priorities, the boards had to take into account the characteristics of their communes, the possibility of implementing these activities in existing conditions. The targets they chose from among the thirty-eight WHO-EURO targets varied, as was expected. Very important has been the role of facilitators in the boards. They have been selected by the project team and their role is to help other group members with knowledge, experience and by disseminating information. They transfer information in both directions and they represent the link between the project team and the territorial health promoting boards.

Thematic groups

Thematic groups are a way to enable the participation of interested citizens in specific matters (priority public health problems and vulnerable groups). So far, we have formed twenty-one such groups, for example:

1 child health
2 adolescent health
3 the health of elderly people
4 a group for the quality of life of disabled people
5 AIDS and STD (sexually transmitted diseases)
6 a group for mental health
7 a group for physical activities
8 group for ecology, and the environment.

These groups work intersectorally with the active participation of professionals and volunteers. Their main tasks are:

1 to determine what resources they have as a group
2 to define the field and targets of work
3 to understand the situation at the city level in relation to the problem
4 to collect present experiences in solving such problems (through models of good practice)
5 to provide a plan and a timetable of activities
6 to develop models for evaluation of their work
7 to define what international activities they could follow and with whom they could collaborate.

The same role which facilitators have on their boards, the moderators play in the thematic groups. Mostly there are two moderators for each group, a professional and a volunteer with experience in that field. The heterogeneous structure of the groups enables wide intersectoral collaboration, exchange of experience and knowledge.

Project function – communication network

There are two communication systems in the project. The central system consists of a network of facilitators (territorial health promoting boards), moderators (thematic groups) and the project team (representatives from the project institutions). Through this network information flows in several ways:

1 by consultation meetings
2 by the distribution of periodicals
3 on the basis of joint information (models of good practice and the production of a Healthy Cities directory)
4 by education seminars.

The broader communication system includes citizens, by opening up the possibilities for individual and group participation in the project. This communication is possible through

1 Healthy Cities mailing boxes placed in prominent public places
2 Local and mass media
3 Printed materials (pamphlets, booklets, leaflets)
4 Exhibitions
5 Telephone hot lines
6 Project institutions
7 Direct contact.

Conclusion

In the past few years Yugoslavia has been going through serious social tensions and deep political crises, putting political conflicts and the fight between different interest groups at the centre of public attention.[1] Health, in a wider social context of uncertainty and fear, has become less interesting than the daily political news. Despite these facts, the evaluation of the project for the past year is positive. The reason why the project is growing in such unpleasant circumstances is because it is widely based on citizens themselves. In everyday living the citizens are faced with many problems which they want to solve to improve their own quality of living.

Of fourteen health promoting boards thirteen are still working, some with more and some with less enthusiasm. The thematic groups are working as well, especially those engaged with the problems of less privileged groups (e.g. the quality of life of people with special needs, elderly people, children, etc.). That has resulted in a joint programme and the founding of a Social Alliance. Ecological groups are becoming stronger and the political changes have introduced new associations such as Green Action, the Union of the Green of Croatia, and so on. The idea of the Healthy Cities is also spreading through Yugoslavia, and we have now established a Yugoslav Healthy Cities network including several cities (Subotica, Dubrovnik, Ljubljana, Split, Osijek, Rijeka).

The social front

A movement under the name of 'Healthy City' has been started in Zagreb with the aim of improving the quality of life in the city (healthy environment, physical and mental health). Within this movement, the idea has been born to organize the activities of those individuals who are, for various reasons, dependent on external help (organized through social work and humanitarian organizations, or spontaneously) to act for themselves and try to solve their own problems. The support they get from the community should be such as to raise their self-esteem rather then make them feel helpless.

The idea was spontaneously given the name 'Social Front' though there are attempts to find a more adequate name for this movement of citizens active in the area of social work and based on the essential values of human beings as individuals and at the centre of communal life – individuals who need and have the right to their own feelings of freedom and justice, the ability to run their own lives, solidarity, equality and so on.

The Social Front is not a political party with a programme to be implemented when it comes to power. Its objectives are to point to the difficulties and to their possible solutions, and to work for change, that is improving the rules, regulations and laws that could enable a better life of the underprivileged categories of urban population.

Because of the economic crisis, social problems have become deeper and more serious. These problems have the greatest impact on the quality of life of the most underprivileged groups of citizens. According to official estimates for March 1990, there are 60,000 subtenants, 80,000 disabled, 130,000 retired, 20,000 unemployed, 50,000 people living on social welfare and other underprivileged groups among the 900,000 inhabitants of Zagreb. There are no reliable data on the exact number of the socially deprived and underprivileged citizens because the town district authorities keep records in a way that does not give a real picture of the situation. The very fact that there are no exact numerical indicators makes it impossible to respond in an adequate manner.

This disintegrated system makes it necessary to create a public atmosphere and stimulate the capabilities of individuals to bring about changes that will contribute to their independence and ability to solve their own problems or to influence the attitudes to the solving of these problems. The basis of the action is support, rather than help through the present social welfare system (as a state body).

While gathering supporters for the Social Front ideas, it was found necessary to train a small group of activists who could act and carry out the set tasks successfully. By applying methods for solving problems of great complexity, diversity and unpredictability (Gaming/Simulation) we can determine the adverse factors that affect the quality of life of the inhabitants of Zagreb and define the methods and scheme of actions. The profusion of obtained ideas and suggestions were synthesized into the Social Front Programme.

The Social Front supports new forms of self-organization, voluntary work and citizens' initiatives. Its programme points to the need for:

1 better informing by establishing an information system and by using mass media, as well as through voting power
2 making a codex of citizens' behaviour
3 implementing a number of changes in the systems of housing, education, social work, transport, nutrition and the like.

Although the Social Front has been functioning for several months, it has already initiated some global and individual actions. Among one of the many global actions going on is the support given to retired persons at risk, giving them so much needed information about credits, ensuring food and ready meals for them. The Social Front has also succeeded in stopping the demolition of temporary shacks for workers and enforced some changes in the law.

Within the frame of the Social Front there exists the Association of Subtenants and the Homeless, which has already established a commission for economic relationships for finding ways of financing future housing construction for homeless people. It has also established a legal counselling service for homeless people and subtenants and has drawn up a project for a future settlement for homeless people.

The Social Front also carries out individual actions, for example to help a disabled person to enter his apartment after seven years of insuperable barriers for him, or to try to solve the health and social problems of a homeless family, such as by the provision of free kindergartens, finding accommodation, and so on. These are only some of the many similar examples of the role of the Social Front.

Participation of the following population groups in the work of the Social Front (since September 1989) has been specially noteworthy:

1 subtenants and homeless people
2 unemployed people
3 disabled people
4 the retired living on small pensions.

Expert associates of the Social Front represent the following organizations: the Red Cross, Caritas, Social Welfare, Employment Agency, mass media, Association of the Disabled, Women's Conference, Green Action, civic authorities, Transcendental Meditation Society, Mountaineering Society, physicians, social workers and others.

Recognizing the benefits of such an organization, it is planned that the Social Front should be registered as a social organization in accordance with legal regulations. This could not have been done before but is possible now that the needs, objectives and potentials have been defined.

Note

1 Since the Zagreb chapter was written events have taken a serious turn for the worse in Yugoslavia. The potential for mutual destruction arising from base inter-communal hatred was anticipated by Slobodan Lang and many others and it prompted the drafting of the following statement on the importance of tolerance and reconciliation as the spiritual prerequisites to health. This statement was submitted to and accepted by the delegates to the 1990 European Healthy Cities Conference in Stockholm.

TOLERANCE AND RECONCILIATION
THE SPIRITUAL PREREQUISITES TO HEALTH

Tolerance is the most important consequence of education: in earlier times people fought for and died for their convictions, but many centuries had to pass by before they understood another form of courage; that is – to recognize the convictions of their close ones and their right to the freedom of conscience. Tolerance is the highest law of each community and it is that spiritual factor which protects all that is best in the thinking of people. No loss from flood, no fire, neither destruction of cities and churches by the inimical forces of nature – has not robbed humanity from so many noble lives and intentions as it was destroyed by mutual intolerance.

Helen Keller (*Optimizam*, 1931)

Hate is the biggest danger to health and the quality of life. Health workers and health services of all countries and in all communities have the responsibility to inform people about the health consequences of hate and to stimulate them to tolerance and reconciliation – reconciliation is also needed between people and the natural environments to which they owe their sustenance.

Any analysis of our world today shows the enormous presence and spread of hatred as a major force of destruction, suffering and death. It also shows how weak is the ability of the health and other sectors to cure hatred once it has been unleashed. If hatred grows even further, the gap between needs and possibilities for health will grow.

Hate is the most dangerous inner pollution; it is the pollution of the spirit.

Hate can take different forms, hatred in the family through the abuse of children, women and old people, as hatred and abuse of other people because of their political or religious beliefs, because of their race, nationality, physical or medical condition or as universal hate of others. Tolerance towards everybody is the most important spiritual prerequisite to health.

Health workers individually, through health services and organizations have a prime duty and responsibility to spread tolerance and do all that is possible to prevent and combat hatred in any form it manifests itself and to work towards reconciliation.

Tolerance is not just the absence of hate. Tolerance is a positive inner, spiritual feeling of security, a desire and willingness to live in peace with all people. Freedom, democracy, human rights, respect, justice, solidarity and reconciliation are the tools evaluating our social relations, inner spirit and consciousness. They are mutually dependent and supportive. Nowhere can tolerance be developed for all times. Everybody should develop, promote, practice, cherish and sustain tolerance. Tolerance includes respect and support for all in freely choosing and living their own way of life. Tolerance also includes cooperation among groups and nations based on the principles of equity, solidarity and respect for all.

References

Adelaide recommendations (1988) Report on the Adelaide conference, Adelaide.

Ashton, J. (1988) 'Tying Down the Indicators and Targets for Health for All', *Community Health Studies* 12: 376–85.

Ashton, J. (1989) *Creating the New Public Health*, WHO Healthy Cities Papers no. 4, Copenhagen: FADL.

Ashton, J. and Seymour, H. (1988) *The New Public Health*, Milton Keynes: Open University Press.

Ashton, J., Grey, P. and Barnard, K. (1986) 'Healthy cities: WHO's new public health initiative', *Health Promotion* 1: 319–23.

Baum, F. and Brown, V.A. (1989) 'Healthy Cities (Australia) Project: Issues of Evaluation for the New Public Health', *Community Health Studies* 13: 140–8.

Brenslow, L. (1989) 'Health Status Measurement in the Evaluation of Health Promotion', *Medical Care* 27/Suppl: S205–216.

Healthy Cities (1988) Zagreb Symposium, Zagreb, vol. 1–3, Zagreb (s.n.).

Kickbusch, I. (1989) *The New Public Health Orientation for the City*, WHO Healthy Cities Papers no. 4, Copenhagen: FADL.

WHO (World Health Organization) (1981) *Global Strategy for Health for All by the Year 2000*, Geneva: WHO.

WHO (1984) *Health Promotion: A Discussion Document on the Concepts and Principles*, Copenhagen: WHO, EURO.

WHO (1985) *Targets in Support of the European Strategy for Health for All*, Geneva: WHO.

WHO (1988) *Leadership Development for Health for All from Alma-Ata to the Year 2000*, WHO resolution WHO 41.26, Geneva: World Health Organization.

Contact

In this chapter we described the Zagreb Healthy City Model, its organization and activities. We have shown only one of the initiatives related to the improvement of quality of life of groups in this city to whom little attention has been paid until now. If you wish to have more information about the Zagreb models of good practice please contact

Dr Selma Ogori
Andrija Tampar School of Public Health
41000 ZAGREB, Rockefellerova 4
Yugoslavia

IV

North American case studies

19

Toronto

Trevor Hancock

The origins of the Healthy City Project in Toronto were described in Chapter 5. In this chapter, I want to describe the evolution of the project and end by speculating on some of the future directions for the project and its implications for city government. But first it is necessary to know something about Toronto.

Toronto

Toronto is Canada's largest city and is located on the northern shores of Lake Ontario, amidst some of the best agricultural land in Canada. It is the capital of Ontario, Canada's most populous province, and the country's industrial heartland and economic powerhouse. Toronto is the economic and communications 'capital' of the country. The city was established in the eighteenth century by British immigrants and was a rather provincial and very 'British' city until after the Second World War; in fact, it was known as 'Toronto the Good'. Since that time the city has grown dramatically and become very cosmopolitan. The original City of Toronto (where the Healthy City Project is located), with its population of 600,000, is now the central core of Metropolitan Toronto, a regional government established in 1953 with six local cities (of which the city itself is one) and a population now grown to 2.2 million. But Toronto has in fact grown well beyond even its metropolitan boundaries, and is now the centre of a Greater Toronto region of some 3.5 million people.

The inhabitants are from all corners of the world, making Toronto one of the most culturally diverse cities to be found anywhere. Roughly half the population have neither English nor French (Canada's two official languages) as their mother tongues and some thirty languages are taught in 'heritage language' classes and used on a daily basis in local press, radio and television media.

For such a large and ethnically diverse city, Toronto has been quite a success story, on the whole, and especially in comparison with cities in the United States. It has a reputation for being clean and safe, for having the best transit system in North America and for having maintained a vibrant and liveable downtown area while preserving its neighbourhoods. Crime rates are low in comparison with the USA (although high in comparison to Europe) and there is not a great deal of ethnic tension; on the whole Toronto celebrates its ethnic diversity and encourages community participation. This has resulted in Toronto being dubbed 'the city that works' and 'a liveable city' and has led the city to develop pretensions to being a world-class city: recently Toronto has been strongly in the bidding for both the 1996 Olympics and Expo 2000.

However, while this is a generally rosy picture, there is another side to the story, in part a consequence of the city's growth and prosperity – what one might call the failure of success. The most obvious area of concern is that of poverty, homelessness and hunger (there is, however, little unemployment). Toronto is now a very expensive city to live in, while minimum wage and social assistance levels have declined in value. As a result, there is a severe shortage of affordable housing and the high cost of housing has meant that many people (perhaps as many as one in twenty, and half of them children) have to resort to food banks regularly: since they first reappeared during the recession of the early 1980s they have become a fixture of city life. Large numbers of people – estimated to be 10,000 to 30,000 – are homeless and living in hostels, and many more are living in very unsatisfactory conditions (Dept Public Health 1988).

The city's physical environment also has problems. There has been extensive development – many would say overdevelopment – of office towers downtown with resultant increases in traffic, while the subway and transit system has not been significantly expanded for some years. Air quality, while generally satisfactory, could be better and the Lake is polluted with chemicals (some fish are not safe to eat) while the beaches are often closed in summer because of sewage pollution (Dept Public Health 1988).

While health and social services are generally of high quality (Canada has universal health insurance and a fairly extensive welfare state) health services are heavily hospital based, and social services create dependency rather than autonomy. Violent crime and crime against women has risen lately, there are of course prostitutes (male and female) and street kids, and cocaine abuse is a growing problem (Dept Public Health 1988).

It is in the context of these successes and the warning signs of failure that the City of Toronto's Healthy Cities Project has developed since 1984.

The Toronto Healthy City Project

It is important to understand first of all that the Healthy City Project is a project of the City of Toronto, the inner urban area of 600,000, and not of Metropolitan Toronto. This is because public health in Toronto is a responsibility of each of the six smaller municipalities, each of which has its own Board of Health, Department of Public Health and Medical Officer of Health. The local municipalities (ranging in size from 600,000 down to 100,000) have their own directly elected Council and Mayor, and are responsible for planning and development, public works, public health, some social housing, parks, buildings inspection and fire services. Metropolitan Toronto, which also has a directly elected Council, is responsible for major parks, roads and planning decisions, the transit system, police, ambulance, social services, some social housing, main sewers and water supply systems. It is also worth bearing in mind that the City of Toronto has a staff of over 6,000 people, and thus is a large and somewhat cumbersome bureaucracy to mobilize.

Health services, it should be added, are not responsible to local government at all, except for public health. In Canada, physicians are mostly private fee-for-service entrepreneurs (except that they bill the government) while hospitals are government-funded but independent non-profit entities. In Metro Toronto, a District Health Council appointed by the provincial government attempts to co-ordinate health care planning, but has no executive authority.

The origins of the Healthy City Project in the report *Public Health in the 1980's*, the subsequent work of the Health Advocacy Unit and the 1984 workshop on *Healthy Toronto 2000* have already been described. Following that workshop, there was a hiatus, due perhaps to the Public Health Department's preoccupation with the ongoing review and renewal of its work stemming from the 1982 reorganization. However, the development of the WHO Healthy Cities Project in Europe spurred – some might say embarrassed – the Board of Health to action. A strategic planning committee established in 1986 began the process of developing an overall strategy to make Toronto a more healthy city. The committee went through a process that included vision workshops with Department staff and community members, a comprehensive environmental scan, the development of an issues paper that was widely distributed in the community, public review and hearings, the development of a final report outlining major issues, strategic mission and priorities and recommendations for action. This process took two years and the final report – *Healthy Toronto 2000* – was approved by the Board of Health in late 1988 and unanimously by City Council in early 1989.

Healthy Toronto 2000, it must be remembered, is a report of the Board of Health, which has responsibility only for the Department of Public Health. However, the report recognizes that 'making Toronto the healthiest city possible' is a task far greater than the Public Health Department could hope to achieve alone. Instead, it requires the combined efforts of all the other Departments of City government, the community (including the business and voluntary sectors) and higher levels of government, notably Metropolitan Toronto.

Accordingly, the report recommends two parallel strategies, the first for the city as a whole, the second for the Department of Public Health. For each strategy, a set of health goals is identified. For the overall Healthy City strategy they are:

1 reduce inequities in health opportunities in Toronto
2 create physical environments supportive of health
3 create social environments supportive of health
4 advocate for a community-based health services system.

These goals deliberately reflect both the *Ottawa Charter for Health Promotion* (WHO *et al.* 1986) and the health goals recommended for the Province of Ontario by a blue-ribbon panel in 1987. Thus the city's health strategy is shown to be related to major international and provincial initiatives, which strengthens its legitimacy and relevance.

The health goals for the Department of Public Health are intended to strengthen the Department's specific role within the broader city-wide initiative. Thus, the goals reinforce the Department's current activities and the traditional public health functions of disease prevention, health protection, health promotion, health education and the collection and analysis of health information. The Department's health goals are as follows:

1 increase health expectancy among the people of Toronto
2 create healthful environments and protect the people of Toronto from health hazards
3 enable the people of Toronto to develop health promotion skills and achieve their health potential
4 plan for health and provide health data for the people of Toronto
5 promote and foster the Healthy City Initiative in all aspects of city life and government.

These health goals are consistent with the new directions established for the Department in the early 1980s, and reinforce many of the innovative programmes the Department has developed during the 1980s, some of which are described below in more detail.

In addition, the report notes three priority principles that should apply to all departmental programmes and to the overall Healthy City initiative. They are based in key social realities of the city, in that they:

1 require that all programmes pay particular attention to the needs of the most disadvantaged and vulnerable groups in the city who experience the greatest inequalities in health
2 emphasize the need for all programmes to recognize the multicultural nature of Toronto and ensure that programmes and activities are socially and culturally appropriate and relevant
3 recommend a community development approach be used in all pro-

grammes in an effort to facilitate the strengthening and empowerment of the community.

Department of Public Health Programmes for a Healthy City

There is neither time nor need to go into the details of public health programmes in Toronto, since the main emphasis of this chapter, and indeed of this whole book, is on the broader approach of the Healthy City Project. However, a number of innovative Public Health Department programmes are of particular relevance to the overall Healthy City strategy. Perhaps chief among those is the Environmental Protection Office (EPO) established in 1986–7.

The EPO resulted from the competition between the incumbent Mayor and a former Board of Health chairwoman who challenged him in 1986. The city's environment became an important campaign issue and each tried to outbid the other to be the best environmentalist. The incumbent Mayor pledged that if he was re-elected he would put in place Canada's first municipal Environmental Protection Office; when he was re-elected he did just that. The EPO is based upon the former health protection section of the Department of Public Health and thus reports through the Medical Officer of Health to the Board of Health. However, it was established under the guidance of a multidepartmental steering group and has a broad responsibility for health protection and environmental quality. Its staff of some fifteen people includes researchers, a toxicologist, an epidemiologist, an urban planner and an environmental health educator. The office has a role in assessing the health implications of major urban planning and development decisions, in investigating environmental contaminants and the threat they pose to human health and assessing threats to Toronto's environmental quality, as well as educating the people of the city about environmental and health concerns. Its reports and recommendations affect the work of many departments and agencies not only in city government but also at metropolitan, provincial, federal and even international levels.

A second important departmental initiative has been the development of by-laws regulating smoking. The first by-law, preventing smoking in public places, was passed in the 1970s. Throughout the 1980s, public pressure and departmental action had seen the by-laws progressively toughened to include a broader range of public spaces, restaurants (which must provide at least 40 per cent non-smoking seating) and most recently the city's work-places. This last by-law is based upon the highly successful San Francisco by-law, in that it does not prohibit smoking but rather it requires that every work-place in the city have a smoking policy in place. The sting is that the smoking policy must be acceptable to the non-smokers in the work-place. The by-law has been widely accepted not only by non-smokers but also by a significant proportion of smokers, who recognized that it may help them to give up, and by employers, who recognize the health, productivity and maintenance cost benefits of a non-smoking work-force. The by-law was accompanied by a major educational campaign, the provision of resource kits to help work-places develop a smoking policy and a troubleshooting and mediation team that would help work-places resolve problems and conflicts. The by-law has been well accepted and remarkably free of trouble, with hardly any cases ending up in court.

The consequence of these non-smoking by-laws and related actions (the public transit system has never allowed smoking, while the Board of Education has virtually prohibited smoking in Toronto's schools) is that many Torontonians live an almost entirely smoke-free existence and smoking has come to be seen as socially unacceptable, which is probably the best way to end the habit.

A third important public health initiative has been in the realm of antenatal education and care and parenting among high-risk groups. For some years, the city's Public Health Department joined with the other Public Health Departments in Metro in funding a Metro-wide antenatal education programme. However, concerned that the programme was failing to reach young, low-income, immigrant and other high-risk groups, the department pulled out of the Metro-wide programme in the mid-1980s and established its own programme, which is designed to reach high-risk, hard-to-reach groups with socially and culturally appropriate programmes and more emphasis on one-to-one rather then group contact. This incorporates lessons learned from two other high-risk maternal and child health programmes.

First, *Healthiest Babies Possible* is an intensive antenatal education and nutritional supplementation programme for pregnant women identified by health and social agencies as high-risk. The programme involves intensive contact and follow-up coupled with food supplementation and has been successful in reducing the incidence of low-birth-weight babies among its recipients.

Second, a similar programme is called *Parents Helping Parents*. In this programme parents identified as at high risk for child neglect or abuse are linked up with specially trained health workers from their own sociocultural groups, who help them cope with the problems of parenting in stressful situations. The programme has the added advantage that it employs and trains women from these disadvantaged communities, providing them with new skills, a useful role in their communities, a sense of self-esteem and the benefit of additional income.

In these and many other innovative ways, the Department of Public Health is fulfilling an important role in helping to make Toronto a more healthy city. In addition, the department pursues its fifth goal of supporting the city-wide Healthy City initiative. It does so primarily through its role in stimulating the creation of the Healthy City Office and in supporting that office, and in working with a variety of agencies and community organizations at the Metro level to try to create a Metro-wide 'healthy community' movement.

The Healthy City Office

The work to establish the city-wide Healthy City initiative begân in parallel with the first work on the *Healthy Toronto 2000* report (1988). An informal group of senior staff from a number of different city departments was brought together in 1986 to begin to explore the Healthy City concepts and its utility to the city. These individuals were hand-picked on the basis of their likely sympathy with the concept, their capacity for innovation and their ability to act as 'champions' for the concept within their own department.

Over a period of a year, they gradually developed a proposal for a formal multidepartmental group with a mandate to hold a series of consultations and vision workshops with staff from all city departments. In particular, the proposal recommended that the multidepartmental group be chaired jointly by the Planning Department and the Department of Management Services. This proposal was approved by the city's 'committee of Heads' (department heads or commissioners) and the proposal was implemented under the leadership of these two departments. Following this, a report on the consultation was sent to the Committee of Heads together with a re-commendation for a city-wide multidepartmental Healthy City Initiative. Two themes were proposed for this initiative, namely urban ecosystem management and social equity. It was also suggested that a further report out-lining the budget and personnel requirements for such an initiative be pre-pared. The report on the consultation was approved, and forwarded to the City Council for information.

It is important to note that to this point, some two years into the process, the Committee of Heads had been asked for little specific commitment except in principle, and City Council had merely been informed but no political approval sought (none being needed, since no new budget requirements were necessary). At the same time, however, the *Healthy Toronto 2000* report, with its eighty-nine recommendations – including one to establish a Healthy City Office – was nearing completion, and was subsequently approved by the Board of Health in late 1988 and unanimously approved by City Council early in 1989. This removed the political uncertainty which had at one point surrounded the *Healthy Toronto 2000* report and had led the multidepart-ment work-group to hesitate to link their proposal too closely to the *Healthy Toronto 2000* report.

As a consequence, it became politically feasible for the multi-department Healthy City work-group to propose in its report to the Committee of Heads a much more ambitious proposal than had originally been envisaged, in-volving a three-person Healthy City Office, a substantial commitment of resources (roughly C$250,000 pa) and a comprehensive strategy of com-munity consultation, information dissemination, information collection, research and analysis. Furthermore, it was clear to the Committee of Heads that such a proposal would be met with strong political support and would enable them to be seen to be leading the initiative.

Thus a Healthy City Office was approved by city council in May 1989 and began operation shortly thereafter. The office is staffed by a manager, a research assistant and a secretary, with a planned expansion in the second year of operation to include a community worker. In accordance with the strategy developed by the interdepartmental steering group and approved by the Committee of Heads and City Council, the office is pursuing three strategies through three subcommittees: communications, project development, and research and analysis.

The first strategy is communications: there are two target populations: the staff of city government and the rest of the population. The former group was identified as a priority for two reasons: first, the need to report back on the progress of the project as a follow-up to the initial consultations and vision workshops conducted a year or two before, and second, the need to ensure that the staff are briefed and educated and prepared to respond to the demands from the community that are likely to follow the community consultation. Staff education has included briefings to the senior management of all departments and a special eight-page edition of the City Hall newsletter. In addition, there are plans for a display highlighting how different departments contribute to the city's health.

Plans for community consultation include a flier to be distributed to every household in the city, a contest to design a logo for the project and community forums and vision workshops to identify community concerns and possible local projects. It is hoped that community grants will then be made available to groups undertaking Healthy City Projects.

The second strategy is project development. Here, the Healthy City Project (HCP) may play several roles. In some instances, it will work with existing City projects that are closely related to the Healthy City concept and could benefit from the injection of Healthy City ideas. Thus the HCP will work with the Food Council recently established by the Board of Health, the Safe City Committee, with a recent 'Green Cities' project and with the 'Mainstreet' project, which is seeking ways to intensify residential density along commercial strips. In addition, the HCP is providing important input to the revision of the Central Area Plan and to major urban housing development projects.

Another role the HCP plays is to initiate or take the lead in specific Healthy City Projects. The most noteworthy of these to date is its role in chairing a new project intended to reduce car use in the city and thus to reduce air and noise pollution. A number of other projects are now under consideration as HCP initiatives.

The third strategy for the HCP is research and analysis. This involves identifying existing data on the health, social and environmental conditions of the city and preparing a 'State of the City' report. The intention is that this will be produced every three years, at the beginning of each new Council term, to provide a basis for each Council's work. The report will be greatly aided by the Department of Public Health's Community Health Survey, produced every five years (most recently in 1989) and a special report on health inequalities to be published in 1990, as well as information assembled for the review of the Central Area Plan and a 'State of the Environment' report published by the EPO in 1988.

A second important task in the area of research and analysis is the development of a monitoring system, including Healthy City indicators to track the project's progress. As other cities have discovered, the development of indicators is a difficult task, and the subcommittee is working with a consultant with a view to following similar developments elsewhere in Canada and the USA.

Implications for the future

As should be clear by now, although the Healthy City Project has been underway in Toronto since 1986, progress is slow. This is not surprising: as is the case elsewhere, smaller cities and towns are able to move much more rapidly to develop and implement an HCP because of the small size and relative intimacy of their decision-making processes and their close and comprehensive community networks. In larger cities, these processes are more cumbersome, more remote, more extensive, more complex and thus more difficult to move.

The slow beginning is not a cause for concern, in part because the HCP is a long-term process in which we are trying to change the corporate and community 'culture' with respect to health, a process which may well take twenty to thirty years to complete. Also, it is important, particularly in large and complex organizations, to build a broad base of support before building the project up: a solid foundation will enable us to build better and achieve more eventually.

Of more concern is the lack of direct, political accountability and community involvement. The former is due to the process by which the project developed within city government and the reporting mechanism to the Committee of Heads. This was not helped by the political uncertainty which at one point surrounded the Board of Health's *Healthy Toronto 2000* Project, which made it unwise to establish a political link at that time and to the fact that the only one of the eighty-nine recommendations in the *Healthy Toronto 2000* report that City Council referred back was one to establish a 'Healthy Public Policy' committee. At the time of writing, therefore, the issue of direct political accountability for the HCP is on the back-burner. Clearly, however, the project and City Council itself will have to come to grips with the need for some sort of political accountability, either through a special committee or some other means.

The need for community involvement in the further development of the project is also crucial. There was community consultation in the preparation of the *Healthy Toronto 2000* report, both through community meetings and through the Board of Health's Community Advisory Boards. While there has been no community consultation in developing the Healthy Cities Project and the office, however, the plans for extensive community consultation and the plans for the development and funding of community projects in 1990, as well as the hiring of community workers, should rectify this situation.

Another aspect of community involvement, however, has yet to be addressed and that is the need for a truly intersectoral (as opposed to interdepartmental) Healthy City Project Committee. A number of key players *beyond* city government are not yet involved in the process. Clearly, a mechanism must be found to involve the business sector, the schools, key voluntary agencies, environmental groups, the health care sector, the churches and other important sectors in developing and guiding the City's Healthy City Project. In addition, there is the challenge already referred to of involving the wider Metro community and government in making the whole of Metro Toronto a more healthy city. This will require forming coalitions with Metro-wide groups and agencies and working to involve Metro Toronto Council and staff in the project.

Let me close with some thoughts about the implications of the HCP for how we organize our city governments. The HCP is one of a number of similar issues – green cities, safe cities, accessible cities and so on – which cut across the traditional and largely nineteenth-century organization of our city government. It is no longer possible, if indeed it ever was, to compartmentalize neatly the city's problems into parks, police, engineering, public health, urban planning and other relatively narrowly defined specialities. The twenty-first century challenges that cities face are holistic and complex in nature, and they require holistic and sophisticated responses. No one group or discipline has the answer, and indeed in working alone they run the danger of only making matters worse. The approach needed now and in the future is for a multidisciplinary and multisectoral approach that combines government, public and private sectors.

One problem is that present city governments are not structured for this holistic approach and have trouble responding to the cross-cutting issues we now face. They will have to adapt, to modify their organizational structure and processes. One way may be to establish a 'matrix-like' structure in which a number of co-ordinators or small offices are responsible for identifying the holistic needs of the city, acting as advocates and co-ordinators within city government and bringing together multidisciplinary and multisectoral work-groups when necessary to address specific issues.

We might then envisage, for example, a Healthy City office with co-ordinators in such areas as social justice, environmental quality, human development, energy and resource conservation/sustainable development, mobility/accessibility and similar areas. Certainly, if the Healthy Cities Project works, we should expect to see it have a long-term impact on the way we run our cities and on the quality of life in those cities.

Further reading

Department of Public Health (1988) *Healthy Toronto 2000*, Toronto, Department of Public Health, City of Toronto (7th Floor, East Tower, City Hall, Toronto, Ontario, M5H 2N2).

Hancock, T. (1990) 'From "Public Health in the 1980's" to "Healthy Toronto 2000": The Evolution of Healthy Public Policy in Toronto', in A. Evers, W. Farrant and A. Trojan (eds) *Local Healthy Public Policy*, Boulder, Colorado: Westview Press.

WHO, Health and Welfare Canada, Canadian Public Health Association (1986) *Ottawa Charter for Health Promotion*, Copenhagen: WHO.

20

California

Joseph M. Hafey, Joan M. Twiss
and Lela F. Folkers

History

In 1987 three Californians were inspired by what they saw and heard at the Healthy Cities Symposium in Düsseldorf, Germany. They were impressed by the Healthy Cities model and felt that, with some adaptation, it had tremendous potential for the State of California. Given the large voluntary agency community, the tradition of private sector involvement in local health issues, and the positive environment for health promotion throughout the State, it was believed that a Healthy Cities approach would be successful.

Shortly after the 1987 Symposium, these three individuals organized a group of community health consultants from throughout the State and began to examine the applicability of the Healthy Cities model for California. This multidisciplinary Organizing Group was comprised of people representing academia, local jurisdictions, and state agencies in California. Subsequently, staff was commissioned to make recommendations on project development and implementation. In January 1989 a contract was let by the California Department of Health Services to the Western Consortium for Public Health, a non-profit organization established by the Schools of Public Health at the University of California, Berkeley, and the University of California, Los Angeles, to conduct the state-wide project. The original Organizing Group was expanded to include broader participation from the private sector, elected officials, and the fields of public administration and urban planning. This expanded group, whose membership reflects the geographic and ethnic diversity of the State, is now the project's Steering Committee.

The unique California environment

A key concern of the organizers was to adapt the WHO Healthy City model to the unique environment in California. California is a large and fascinating State that economically ranks as the sixth largest economy in the world. It covers 158,693 square miles and extends approximately 1,000 miles along the Pacific coastline. Its geography is varied including highly urbanized areas, vast open spaces, and large agricultural tracts.

In designing the California Healthy City Program, the Advisory Committee considered the following eight factors.

First, the State's 28 million population is undergoing rapid demographic change. As much as one-third of the total US immigrant population has been settling in California changing the State into a true melting pot of diversified racial and ethnic groups. Hispanics account for 24 per cent of the population, Blacks 7.5 per cent and Asians 8 per cent. Since many of these minority groups are also poor, they bear a disproportionate share of health and societal problems. The combination of poverty and cultural and linguistic barriers poses a real challenge to all institutions in California to find new solutions. Cities are aware and interested in addressing these issues.

Second, there is a great receptivity throughout California towards new approaches to improving health through both individual behaviour modification and institutional change. Characteristically, the Golden State's people are forward thinking, ideas driven, and less bound to traditional methods of problem-solving. Exercise, nutrition, tobacco control, tougher drunk driving laws, injury prevention, AIDS education, self-help, and self-esteem, as well as a widespread environmental protection movement, for example tough vehicle emission standards, carcinogen labelling, and recycling have all become significant trends in California.

Third, many of the State's government organizations have demonstrated tremendous leadership in areas that affect health. The State Department of Health Services initiated the Healthy Cities Project and provides the focus for integrating other State programmes. Together with other State agencies, such as Mental Health, Education, Air Resources, Alcohol and Drugs it has also initiated creative programmes in cancer control, giving up smoking and AIDS education. Each is known for establishing creative new programmes that affect the health of people.

Fourth, California has a rich network of universities that have considerable resources which can assist cities. The Schools of Public Health at the University of California (Berkeley and Los Angeles) and San Diego State University, in particular, have faculty and programmes that can provide technical assistance in almost any problem area. They are major partners in the Healthy Cities Project.

Fifth, cities in California, numbering over 450, are rapidly accepting an expanded role in improving the health and quality of life of their citizens. The size and diversity of these cities and the growth in their sponsorship of Healthy City Projects offer an excellent base to expand and build on the concept. At the 1989 annual meeting of the League of California Cities, almost 25 per cent of the agenda dealt with issues directly related to public health or quality of life.

Sixth, the strong role of county governments in health care, health promotion, and environmental health offers an opportunity to develop county–city partnerships that will extend resources for community improvement. Counties have the opportunity to provide leadership and technical assistance to their cities in improving the quality of life.

Seventh, there is a high level of private and voluntary agency activity in community health that can be harnessed at both the local and State level by the Healthy Cities movement. Large disease-orientated voluntary organizations such as the American Cancer Society and American Heart Association have gradually moved into health policy and promotion. Business is very active in employee health promotion, health care cost containment, and community well-being. Philanthropic foundations are increasingly focusing programmes that are directed at creative community problem-solving and the health care delivery system is increasingly aware of the importance of its involvement in community decision-making. Overall, there is a growing understanding by individual sectors that problems cannot be solved in isolation but require the collaboration of all sectors. Given the ability of cities to organize disparate community groups, they are attractive focal points for this community collaboration around issues such as health which have a direct bearing on individuals' well-being and the viability of all sectors within a community.

Finally, there is a long history and strong tradition of community participation in solving local problems in California. De Tocqueville recognized the propensity of Americans to organize, found new agencies, and to speak out to express their demands for change. The 'Green Movement' to preserve the environment, groups like Mothers Against Drunk Driving and Americans for Nonsmokers' Rights, as well as the active participation of individuals in governmental, civic, fraternal and religious organizations are examples of Californians' receptivity to concepts like Healthy Cities.

The California Healthy Cities Project

The California Healthy Cities Project looks very much like its European WHO predecessor parent. It is built upon the premise of shared responsibility among individuals, the government, and the private sector. Local involvement is the cornerstone of the movement. The project's mission is to reduce inequities in health status that exist between population groups in cities.

The project focuses on the official city government as the most appropriate site for institutionalizing the Healthy Cities concept. Although counties and neighbourhoods were considered, as entities for participation in the project, the decision was made early on to focus the limited available project resources on the official city institution as it appeared most able to draw diverse community groups together while providing an inherent and important sense of ownership for activities.

How cities become participants

A competitive process was designed in which cities were required to submit formal proposals for participation with the expectation that six to eight California cities would be selected. Interested cities were asked to submit ten-page proposals and work plans with the following required information:

1 Provision of a *rationale* as to why the city should be considered for participation, including a description of the city's experience with similar projects.
2 Resolution by the city council, and endorsement by other appropriate community organizations, to participate in the project using a broad public policy approach to health.
3 Description of resources from within the community which will be devoted to the project. Community groups, the private sector or the city administration may wish to contribute time, staff and/or money to their local effort.
4 Provision of an *organizational plan* for identification and prioritization of community needs as well as *how* needs would be addressed.
5 Description of how the various sectors in the community, i.e. public, private and community groups, will be involved in the Healthy Cities process. This would include, at a minimum, participation in a local steering committee. This committee should include persons who can affect changes in community-wide policies and practices as well as those who are affected by them.
6 Description of how the local steering committee would work with the county health department and other local health agencies and organizations.
7 Description of how the project will address issues of equity, that is how the problem/need affects minority populations in the community and how its resolution will positively influence their well-being.
8 Agreement to participate in the *evaluation* of the project both statewide and locally. Suggestions should be provided as to how the local projects might be evaluated.
9 Agreement to share resources, strategies and experiences with projects in other cities and the state-wide project.

What the cities get from the project

In the same way as its European forebear, the California Healthy Cities Project provides no direct financial assistance to the cities. The project does provide for consultants to render on-site technical assistance. It also sponsors training, and brokers' assistance and resources for cities from other public and private programmes throughout the State in such areas as mental health, injury prevention, alcohol and drug prevention, tobacco control, nutrition and cancer control, environmental improvement, and community health promotion. Designated cities also have permission to use the official California Healthy Cities logo.

All cities in the State can take advantage of several project services. A newsletter, information from a computerized database of innovative Healthy Cities-type strategies, state-wide conference opportunities, resource packages, and referral to resources for funding and programme enrichment are all provided without charge to interested cities and public health agencies.

The first seven cities

The level of commitment by the city to the Healthy Cities Project was the key criterion for the selection of cities. When commitment was demonstrated by elected officials, administration, and community groups, it was much more likely that the city's project would be successful. In September 1989 the Project Steering Committee recommended the first five cities for participation and designated two more in January 1990. These cities are Arcata, Bell, Duarte, Long Beach, Palm Desert, Pasadena and South El Monte. The following profiles of the first seven cities highlights their diversity as well as their broad range of projects and varied approaches undertaken by the cities.

Arcata

The City of Arcata is located in Northern California, approximately 300 miles north of San Francisco on Humboldt Bay. It has a total population of 15,000. The combined 6 per cent ethnic minority population breaks down as follows: 3 per cent Native American, 2 per cent Asian, 0.5 per cent Black and 0.4 per cent Hispanic. The remainder of the population is Caucasian. Compared with state-wide averages, Arcata has a high percentage of unmarried people (56 per cent in Arcata, 43 per cent state-wide) a high percentage of people below the poverty level (25 versus 10 per cent); a high percentage of active 15–34-year-old age group (60 versus 37 per cent); and a high percentage of people in rented accommodation (55 versus 45 per cent). This combination creates an unusually high demand for affordable community facilities.

Arcata's project entails building a community centre which will serve as a focal point for community-wide physical and social activities, fostering a sense of well-being and belonging among residents. It is expected to be fully operational within six years. Input regarding needs and opinions concerning the use of the centre, has been gathered from different community groups, such as elderly people, teenagers, parents, pre-school children, and people on low incomes. By the end of the first year, schematic drawings and plans will

21

Indiana

Melinda Rider and Beverly C. Flynn

Introduction

The Healthy Cities Indiana Programme is trying to adapt the European and Canadian Healthy Cities models to cities in the United States. This presents a forceful challenge. Indiana cities, as most cities in the United States, are faced with a series of phenomena which present obstacles to community-wide health promotion. These phenomena include a decentralization and fragmentation of responsibility for the health of citizens from federal to state and local levels of government without accompanying fiscal support; a public health system that, according to the Institute of Medicine (1988) Report, is in disarray; and, a market driven health care system that spends about 95 per cent of the health care dollar on highly technical medical care. Healthy Cities Indiana is, as well, occurring within a system of representative democracy which presents its own unique challenges and opportunities for community-based problem-solving.

Healthy Cities and citizen participation

The concept of Healthy Cities entails a commitment to community involvement in decisions about health. Seen in this light, health becomes part of the civic responsibility of the individual as well as the public responsibility of the government. A major goal of the Healthy Cities movement is to put health on the public agenda and therefore subject to the balancing of interests inherent in any policy arena. Paramount to this balancing of interests, however, is that the *community* interest is well represented. Successful Healthy Cities programmes must therefore take into account the local political culture so that equal interests can be equally represented in the policy process. Healthy Cities Indiana seeks to adapt the European and Canadian models of Healthy Cities to the United States and to Indiana. To do that, the political culture of both the country, the state, and the communities, must be understood.

Background

In the United States local government is traditionally viewed as the 'school room' for democracy. It is at the local level where people are thought to be able to participate most fully in the decisions that directly affect their lives (Bulpit 1972). Because the opportunity for participation is there, and because the link between participation and policy outcome is most clear and most immediate, local politics is the place where citizens 'practise' democracy in order to gain experience, competence, knowledge and efficacy for the ideals of democratic self-government. These experiences with democratic participation at the local level should, it is thought, build within the citizen the ability to move on to the more complex decisions of national government (Pateman 1970).

However, the highly fractionalized system of government in the United States means that decisions are usually made in a series of steps, requiring the attention of the would-be participant in several directions and to differing levels of government. In the United States, therefore, the citizen must not only understand the policy-making process but also be able to bear the costs of participation: time, effort, transportation, technical knowledge and organization. In addition to these difficulties, sometimes the decision-making process is not open nor does it lend itself to disturbances to the status quo. Frequently, therefore, it seems the *difficulty* of participating leads to the *failure* to attempt to participate. Finally, it is not clear that citizen participation is other than a procedural change that does not necessarily lead to policy change. Nevertheless, citizen participation remains a widely-held value in the United States and this is especially true in local areas.

In addition to the value placed on civic responsibility, citizens of the Midwestern area of the United States share a number of other cultural values which have been key in the successful adaptation of the Healthy Cities model. A generally strong work ethic leads these citizens to believe that if the effort and skill are sufficient, the desired result cannot fail but be obtained. A spirit of voluntaryism is also present which encourages people to spend leisure time in efforts which benefit the community. This combination of the work ethic, sense of civic responsibility, and voluntaryism, has led to a belief that the individual *has* a responsibility for the welfare of the community and the individual *can* make an effort which will have an impact upon the community.

Healthy Cities Indiana

Background

Indiana is slightly more rural than the United States as a whole, and education level, income, and living standards lag behind national averages. In the last decade the state's economy has been hit hard by the out-migration of manufacturing jobs, replaced by lower paying, light industry and service-sector employment.

Minorities in Indiana are concentrated in the larger cities with some 92 counties having virtually no minority population. Health status trends have been uneven over the last decade but on nearly every indicator, with the exception of lung diseases, residents of Indiana have poorer health status than the United States as a whole. Infant mortality rates continue to outpace the nation, and in Indianapolis, the state capital, the non-white infant mortality rate frequently leads the nation for cities of its size (in 1986 there were 25.7 deaths per 1,000 live births). While increased access to medical care might ameliorate the worst excesses, dramatic improvements in health status are beyond the reach of the privatized sick care system. What is required are broad-range solutions aimed at multiple, complex problems and involving co-ordinated efforts by the entire community. Solutions will necessarily come from changes in public policies regarding the major health indicators: employment, education, environmental quality, access to appropriate supports for healthy behaviours, and the meeting of basic life requirements.

The question, of course, is how to achieve holistic approaches to improving health status. Based on the belief that improved policies affecting health come about as a result of broad-based community support for change, Healthy Cities Indiana's major goal is to build viable, community-based leadership for promoting healthy public policies. With funding from the Kellogg Foundation and the Indiana University School of Nursing, Healthy Cities Indiana supports community participation in the healthy public policy process by providing technical assistance to build the community competence needed by those citizens who are normally priced out of the policy process. By joining the non-participant with the established order, Healthy Cities Indiana provides a catalyst for community participation in, and control over, decisions which affect health.

Developing Healthy Cities in Indiana

The Indiana University School of Nursing Department of Community Health Nursing has based its graduate degree curricula on the concept of primary health care as developed by the World Health Organization at the Alma Ata Conference in 1978. In keeping with these principles of primary health care – equitable distribution, community involvement, focus on prevention, appropriate technology, and a multisectoral approach – the department sponsors each year a conference aimed at addressing the pressing issues of primary health care. The 1987 conference, 'Health for All by the Year 2000: Progress in the Americas', included a presentation by Dr Trevor Hancock, one of the developers of the WHO Healthy Cities model. In the context of a presentation about Canadian progress toward the Health for All goals, Dr Hancock briefly discussed the Canadian experience with Healthy Cities. From this exposure, Dr Beverly Flynn, began the development of the collaborative project known as Healthy Cities Indiana. This project is based closely on the principles of primary health care as articulated in the Alma Ata statement and taught in the Department of Community Health Nursing at Indiana University since 1978.

Objectives of Healthy Cities Indiana

As in the European model, Healthy Cities Indiana seeks to *put health first* on the political agenda, requiring city policy-makers to consider the health effects of all their decisions. Additionally, Healthy Cities Indiana sees health as a *shared responsibility of the entire community*, not just the health professions. As a shared responsibility, decisions about health should *involve local people* – those whose lives will be affected by these decisions. Involving local people also means *focusing on those people who are hard to reach*: the poor, the homeless, population groups, and the elderly are examples. Finally, by recognizing health as a responsibility of *both* the public and private sectors, Healthy Cities Indiana hopes to *promote healthy public policies* which ensure health for all.

Selection of the participating cities

Using the three regions of the Indiana Public Health Association (north, central, and south), sixteen cities were identified and existing data about these sixteen cities were collected. The criteria for targeting as a participating city in the Healthy Cities Indiana Project were first, the existence of populations at risk to health problems, and second, demonstrated community support for participation in the project. Based on recommendations from local activists with the Indiana Public Health Association, six cities and four alternates, all with populations at risk to health problems, were targeted for approach by the project staff.

Again with the assistance of local public health professionals and selected community leaders, community representatives were identified to attend a presentation about Healthy Cities Indiana. This presentation included a short video introducing the Healthy Cities concept, an explanation of the Healthy Cities Indiana Project (including the costs and benefits of participation to the city), and an open discussion of issues and concerns about the project. In some cities more than one presentation was made, each to a different group of local people. Local support for the project was determined from

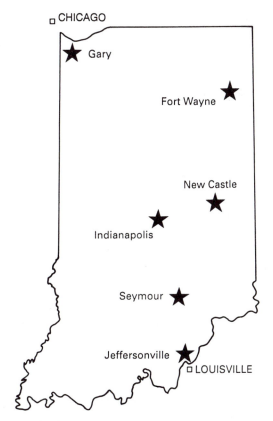

Figure 21.1 A map of Indiana showing the six selected cities.

these initial meetings as well as by the willingness of the mayors and the local health officers to sign a 'memorandum of understanding' indicating their understanding of, and their support for, participation in Healthy Cities Indiana. One of the six targeted cities could not reach a determination of their interest in participation therefore an alternate city in that region was approached and selected. A map of Indiana with the six selected cities appears in Figure 21.1.

The Healthy City Committees

Developing the local Healthy City Committees involved a process of defining categories for representation (see Table 21.1), identifying appropriate local people for those categories, and establishing their interest in, and capacity for, participation. The selection of committee members was an important key to the progress of the project locally. For some cities, settling on a working committee was a difficult process, sometimes taking nearly a year before the committee was fully in place and working smoothly.

Table 21.1 Categories for committee members

Arts and Culture	Health Care Utilities and Energy
Business and Industry	Indiana Public Health Association
Dentistry	Local Government
Education	Media
Employment: Planning and Housing	Parks and Recreation
Environment: Population Groups	Religion
Finance	Transportation and Communication

Another key to the effective functioning of the committees is the strong support of the mayors. In the smaller cities the mayor was a member of the Healthy City Committee while in the larger cities the mayor appointed a staff person to represent his interests. Cities whose mayors took a strong interest in the activities of the local Healthy City Committee progressed more quickly. Clearly some mayors recognized early the political advantage in public support for the Healthy Cities Indiana Project. In every city the local public health professionals have been full participants. Healthy Cities Indiana has proved to be an exciting means of reuniting public health with political processes resulting in increased exposure of public health expertise to the community.

Leadership development

Integral to the success of Healthy Cities Indiana is the development of leaders for health promotion at the local level. Every community has leaders but those outside the traditional health sector often do not realize their potential role in health promotion, and most community leaders lack the diverse range of skills needed for the development of, and effective advocacy for, healthy public policies.

In order to develop leadership for health, annual workshops are held where committee members are taught such skills as utilizing data, meeting skills, working with the media, conducting and analysing community surveys, setting priorities among competing community concerns, finding solutions, and the policy process. Healthy Cities Indiana designed and conducted most of the workshop sessions, bringing in such consultants as Dr Trevor Hancock and Dr John Ashton when additional expertise was needed. These workshops have been developed into modules for use with new cities coming into the programme.

Cognizant of the need for developing a state-wide network for promoting healthy public policies in the Indiana legislature, all six Healthy City Committees meet together annually in sessions designed to provide topical information and to share experiences and expertise. These network sessions provide a sense of vanguardship to the committee members and give them a sometimes needed exhilaration to continue the hard work of building healthy communities. In the second year of the programme, the chairs and co-chairs of the committees formed an advisory group for the Healthy Cities Indiana Programme in order to guide the development of further materials and workshop content. The Kellogg funding also provides for underwriting the cost of committee member attendance at conferences where they can further develop their expertise. This conference attendance was particularly significant after the committees had established their priorities and needed guidance on developing solutions. The materials developed by Healthy Cities Indiana staff are also collected in the Healthy Cities Resource Center located at Indiana University School of Nursing in Indianapolis, Indiana. Finally, Healthy Cities Indiana staff, experienced in community development, are constantly available to local Healthy City Committees to provide assistance.

Community assessment

In each participating city Healthy City Committee members are given a workbook containing existing data about their city: population broken down by age, race and gender; employment statistics; family patterns; educational achievement; infant mortality rates; leading causes of death; crude birth-rates and death-rates; and housing data. Much of these data were presented over time so that major trends could be observed. Each category of data was compared, when possible, to averages for Indiana and the United States so that committee members could see where exceptional divergences from the norm occurred. This workbook also contained a community check-list which helped the committee members to assess various facets of their community. With the assistance of the staff of Healthy Cities Indiana, the committees then began to determine where the gaps in the data lay, and what issues were community problems. The data also helped the committees to identify community strengths and resources.

A few months into the programme most committees began to realize that while they had numbers about their city, they didn't know what the *people* in the community wanted or even thought about. The committees then began in various ways to go about getting what have been referred to as the 'stories' of the community.

The committees were particularly interested in including the youth of their city in their projects and all devised ways to include children in the assessment process: three of the cities used a version of the Seattle KidsPlace survey; one city conducted a city-wide poster competition around the theme 'Vision of a Healthy City' for schoolchildren in grades four to twelve (aged 9–17); one city developed a survey on drug abuse to be used with very young children (grades two and four) (aged 7 and 9); and one city used another version of the KidsPlace survey for both adults and children.

The cities understood the need to include a cross-section of their city in the survey process and at least one took extraordinary steps to be sure that at-risk populations were included by taking their survey to homeless shelters, senior citizen centres, juvenile detention centres and halfway houses for offenders. What the committees learned were the 'stories' of their communities: what the people were concerned about, what they liked about their city, and, what they didn't like.

The Healthy Cities Indiana approach to complex problem-solving

The next step for the local committees was to identify the health problems in their community and the resources available to resolve those problems. Using the existing data compiled by Healthy Cities Indiana staff and the community surveys, the committees were able to come to consensus on both the problems and the priority for those problems. Assessing community strengths helped the committees begin to think about possible solutions to their problems. The Healthy Cities Indiana staff provided technical assistance to the committees by reviewing existing programmes and suggesting potential solutions.

Healthy Cities Indiana asks local communities to assess the health of their community, including both community strengths and weaknesses, and develop action strategies which lead to improvements in health status. However, improvements in the indicators of health status (infant mortality, mortality and morbidity rates, etc.) take a number of years and other aspects of health may not be easily quantifiable. Cities participating in the Healthy Cities Indiana Programme were encouraged both to break complex problems down into components which were not so overwhelming, and to combine short-term projects – with more immediate payoffs – with long-range solutions aimed at policy change. Table 21.2 lists many of the projects, both short-term and long-range, which the cities have undertaken.

Engaging the community in the great debate about health

The community surveys were the first steps in opening up the debate about health to the community. Other means were also used to increase the quantity of discussions: booths at health fairs were used to ask opinions about the local community; the local media were used to spread information about the Healthy Cities Indiana Programme in the local community; vision workshops were conducted with community groups; short-term projects resulted in a raised awareness of the broader definition of health; speakers' bureaux were formed to carry the message into the community. Across the six cities few methods for reaching the broader community went unused.

Analysis of Healthy Cities Indiana

While all members of a community can agree that a Healthy City is in everyone's best interest, how best to achieve health, and at whose expense, are questions that are often quite divisive. By bringing representatives of all the vested interests together, common goals could be established. By

Table 21.2 Examples of local solutions

Short-term actions	Mouth-guard campaign for children in contact sports
	Community walking club
	'Healthy Moments' radio messages
	'Vision of a Healthy City' poster competition
	Family drug education
	City street clean-up
	Health fairs with health screening
Long-range strategies	City-wide kerb-side recycling programme
	Comprehensive teenage–parent education
	Comprehensive solutions for affordable housing shortage
	Developing state legislative commitment to promoting Healthy Cities in Indiana

accepting common – and equal – responsibility for the health of the community, this public–private partnership was able to bypass any placing of blame for current community conditions, and move on to the important work of problem-solving.

The Healthy City Committees in each of the participating cities were quick to see that assessment and planning were key to solving community problems, but that implementation was the critical element often missing in previous community efforts. Every committee could recount numbers of community task forces, or hired expert panels who studied a community problem with great thoroughness, made sometimes cogent recommendations for solutions, but the reports gathered dust in city offices. When the community isn't involved in both the agenda setting *and* the policy formulation stage of the policy process, then ownership is lacking and support for proposed changes does not develop.

Healthy Cities Indiana, in adapting the European and Canadian models to Indiana, has endeavoured to involve the community at every step of the process for developing healthy public policies. People not only define their problems, but also find workable solutions, adequate funding, appropriate techniques for implementation and monitoring results. The existence of the widely held values of self-reliance, local control, and community participation in the political process – while admittedly too seldom acted upon – are clear advantages for positive implementation of Healthy Cities Projects in Indiana. The *authority* of the local citizens to act on their own behalf is supported in law and is generally not questioned. The political systems appear to be open enough to allow broad-based participation, particularly when the advantages of the public–private partnership can be demonstrated to local politicians. Rapid dissemination of Healthy Cities is expected and will be facilitated through the Healthy Cities Indiana Resource Center. In addition, Healthy Cities Indiana and the National League of Cities are co-operating in the dissemination of information about Healthy Cities in the United States in order to reach approximately 16,000 local municipalities associated with the National League of Cities.

204 *Melinda Rider and Beverly C. Flynn*

The success of Healthy Cities Indiana demonstrates the affinity of the social and political culture in the United States to implementation of primary health care in the Alma Ata tradition, and provides a mechanism whereby implementation can take place.

References and further reading

Bulpit, J.G. (1972) 'Participation and Local Government: Territorial democracy', in G. Parry (ed.) *Participation in Politics*, Manchester, Mich: Manchester University Press.

Bureau of the Census (1982) *General Population Characteristics: Indiana*, Washington DC: US Department of Commerce.

Division of Public Health Statistics (1988) *Indiana Health Profile 1988*, Indianapolis: Indiana State Board of Health.

Institute of Medicine (1988) *The Future of Public Health*, Washington, DC: National Academy Press.

Lassey, W.R. and Fernandez, R.R. (1986) *Leadership and Social Change*, La Jolla, California: University Associates.

Parry, G. (ed.) (1972) *Participation in Politics*, Manchester, Mich: Manchester University Press.

Pateman, C. (1970) *Participation and Democratic Theory*, Cambridge: Cambridge University Press.

WHO (World Health Organisation) (1978) *Alma Ata. Primary Health Care*, Geneva: World Health Organization.

WHO, Health and Welfare Canada, Canadian Public Health Association (1986) *Ottawa Charter for Health Promotion*, Copenhagen: World Health Organization, Regional Office for Europe.

V

Antipodean case studies

22

Palmerston North

Janet Takarangi and Hoane Kataka Takarangi

Introduction

New Zealand, Aotearoa, Land of the Long White Cloud, has two beginnings. In the ancient beliefs of the first people of the land (the *tangata whenua*) the Maori, Aotearoa was fished from the ocean depths by Maui. The second beginning is attributed by tradition to Kupe who on a voyage from Hawaiiki discovered Aotearoa about AD925. Waves of canoe fleets from throughout the Pacific followed so that by the time of European colonization in the eighteenth century the people of Aotearoa were the descendants of successive groups of immigrants.

New Zealand's population today is 3.3 million, spread over a land area the same size as the British Isles or Japan. Our cities are small by world standards. New Zealand is currently undergoing a planned economic transformation. This is altering amongst other things urban–rural settlement patterns, social structures, economic production modes and land use. New Zealand and New Zealanders over the last few years have made important international stands on peace, nuclear testing in the South Pacific, driftnet fishing and whaling. These stands have been made by working collaboratively with other nations and with indigenous peoples in the Pacific.

Megatrends down under

The socio-political environment provides a useful context for understanding the Healthy Cities movement in New Zealand. Naisbett (1984) identified ten megatrends that can be used to identify current patterns and changes in New Zealand. New Zealand's economy since the first refrigerated ship carried meat to the United Kingdom in 1892 has been agriculturally based. Produce was exported in bulk and only recently have significant gains been made in developing food processing to add value to our products before export.

The Closer Economic Relations (CER) Trade Pact with Australia signed in 1983 has led to changes in imports, exports and manufacturing patterns. Trade agreements with countries around the Pacific rim as well as New Zealand's traditional trading partners has led to a more dynamic trading mix. Changes in foreign exchange controls have strengthened the country's awareness of being part of a dynamic global economy.

Working to turn economic and traditional expectations around has meant that the emphasis in New Zealand has had to shift from short-term goals (often defined in three-yearly terms to coincide with the national elections) to long-term planning. Economists vary in their views on short-term pain for long-term gain, with 147,866 people unemployed (11.03 per cent of labour force as at February 1990), many New Zealanders can comment personally on the pain (Department of Statistics 1990).

With recent changes in health, education, local government and social welfare areas together with major legislative changes pending for environmental resource management and tribal development for Maori people Naisbett's trends of

- centralization to decentralization
- institutional help to self-help
- representation to participation

are clearly apparent.

Devolution has been the catchword in New Zealand since the mid-1980s. Decentralizing services from national bureaucratic control to enhance local responsiveness and accountability have been the reasons quoted behind the changes. Some sectors such as health (Area Health Boards) and local government (Community Boards, City, District and Regional Councils) have clear legislative mandates for community participation. The National Health Charter released in 1989 identified five key principles:

1 community involvement
2 respect for individual dignity
3 equity of access
4 disease prevention and health promotion
5 effective resource use.

Local government has powerful legal requirements that dictate not only what the community will participate in, but also how. What is clear, is that it will be those organizations which have the ability to think creatively, to be customer orientated, to work from grass-roots up, to develop and maintain effective networks and to generate and consider multiple options for complex issues that will flourish in the current environment.

New Zealand is also going through a change of identity as we move from being a country in the South Pacific to a South Pacific country with our unique history, language and traditions. The Treaty of Waitangi signed in 1840 by agents of the Crown and Maori people as first people of the land is becoming recognized as the country's foundation document. Maori beliefs on health like indigenous peoples elsewhere are linked to the land, the environment, blood ties and ancestry. Maori health is related to the belief that people are part of their environment. The *Whenua* (Land) is seen as the Mother of all life, of *tangata* (people) of trees, birds, and all living things on land and in the oceans. The connection is seen as all important, for without land, people have no foundation to support them.

The Maori of Aotearoa believe their *whakapapa* (genealogy) reaches back to the primeval parents Ranginui the Sky Father and Papatuanuku the Earth Mother. This belief that Land, sky and people are part of each other is the basis of health for Maori people. Thus, there is rejection of the artificial divisions created between mind, body and spirit by Western medicine. These beliefs are starting to be acknowledged in how health services are delivered in New Zealand and agencies are being challenged to be more holistic in how they develop their role in society. Healthy Cities as a concept is compatible with this changing view of health in New Zealand, a view that demands and acknowledges multiple answers to health questions.

Healthy Cities: gathering momentum in New Zealand

John Ashton's visit to New Zealand in 1988 was timed to capture the energy and interest being expressed within health and other sectors for new ways of doing things. Primary health care, the Alma Ata Declaration (WHO 1978) and the Ottawa Charter (WHO *et al.* 1986) had been embraced by people but it was an uphill battle to make it real. Healthy Cities offered an opportunity to take primary health care 'off the shelves and into the streets and communities' of New Zealand and to build on the gathering global energy for change.

Throughout the country people picked up ideas from the Ashton presentations and so the movement spread to New Zealand. Since 1988 as Healthy Cities has been introduced various initiatives have commenced, each one different, each one reflective of the people, community and agencies involved. There are now projects in Manukau City Auckland, Palmerston North, Lower Hutt City, Wellington City, Christchurch, and a Healthy Communities project in Otago.

The following case studies reflect this dynamic process.

Healthy City: Lower Hutt

Lower Hutt Healthy Cities is based on the co-operative approach, encouraging community involvement and co-operation between sectors to create positive health environments. Following the New Zealand Public Health

Association (NZPHA) Healthy Cities Conference in May 1988, the Healthy Cities approach was identified as an action-based strategy towards achieving 'Health for All by the Year 2000' based on the Ottawa Charter:

1 building healthy public policy
2 creating supportive environments
3 strengthening community action
4 developing personal skills
5 reorientating health services.

The Lower Hutt Health Development Unit (the regional office of the Department of Health, now with the Wellington Area Health Board) along with the Lower Hutt City Council, resolved in 1988 to actively support the establishment of an intersectoral Healthy Cities Committee.

In December 1988, having recognized that the Healthy Cities concept and urban planning are essentially concerned with social and economic well being, Council resolved that

The Healthy Cities concept be incorporated into the development and implementation of the City Centre Urban Structure Plan and other council projects.

The Health Development Unit demonstrated their commitment to Healthy Cities by strengthening working links with the Council. Placement of a staff member with the Council's Community Development Division helped to forge and strengthen networking and demonstrate new ways of working in Lower Hutt. Two major workshops led to the establishment of the Lower Hutt Healthy Cities Core Group representing local authority, central government and community organizations. Participants at the workshops consistently identified effective communication and co-ordination between sectors, along with getting professionals 'on tap and not on top' as being necessary to achieve health goals.

Health promotion issues are discussed at regular well-supported Core Group meetings, workloads are shared and a person elected by the group acts as co-ordinator thus providing a consistent point of contact. The Healthy Cities Co-ordinator has been responsible for starting a national newsletter and hosting a national meeting designed to strengthen networks.

Posters, supplements in the local newspaper and a Healthy Cities floral garden were promotional activities used to raise public awareness of the project in Lower Hutt. The Lower Hutt Healthy Cities logo encourages local identification with an international project combining a local flavour of hills and trees with the World Health Organization's strategy of 'Health for All by the Year 2000'.

Re-establishment of a community newsletter, generating broad-based support for projects such as safety helmets for cyclists and safe cycleways, purchasing and running a Healthy Cities van are some of the activities undertaken by the Core Group. The van illustrates the Healthy Cities approach in action. Mechanical expertise and garaging was provided by local police, van seating by the Health Development Unit and new tyres by anonymous donations. A NZ$10,000 grant from the Council provided the base funding. A Restart worker (a Labour Department initiative for employment) organizes the daily running, administration and bookings for the van. By combining skills and resources, the Healthy Cities Core Group was able to achieve what no one group had been able to do alone, keeping the cost for users to a minimum. The Healthy Cities van sporting the logo is in demand by community groups helping to meet a deficiency in transport availability especially for adolescents and elderly people. A community health project in a large state housing development illustrates further the benefits of joint action. The residents now have access to a community house which they run and which caters to their social needs. The house is leased from the city council on land donated by the Housing Corporation. This initiative involved local health workers, Members of Parliament, the Wellington School of Medicine and numerous workers from other agencies.

Healthy Communities: Otago

Formed in May 1988 the Action Group of volunteers has increased its network and is making steady progress. A set of objectives for 1989 saw the development of a Starter Resource Kit including a first attempt at a community diagnosis based on health indicators. This kit was 'launched' at a public seminar in 1989. Involvement of local politicians, key opinion-makers and a wide range of community and statutory groups working together to raise awareness of health has been part of the plan. The logo, designed by a talented young person from the area, reflects Otago's approach to the international movement.

Local government reorganization on a large scale has resulted since October 1989 in regional and local councils as well as community boards being established. New boundaries, functions and pending legislation have provided the Action group and its members with new opportunities to be involved in shaping the political agenda. Candidates standing for the election to local government were sent the seminar reports, those successfully elected were sent full kits. The emphasis was on developing the idea of healthy public policy and on showing how attitudes can affect health through decisions made by community leaders. Since the elections the Regional Council for Otago and the Dunedin City Council have had agenda items on the philosophy and objectives of Healthy Communities Otago. The Dunedin City Council Initiatives Committee has lent its support to the establishment of a regional committee on public health.

The Action group with its increasing network of contacts has drawn up objectives for 1990. Housing will be a key focus. Affordable housing, housing for older people and the state of the housing stock will be discussed. The Action group is supported by staff from the Otago Area Health Board and the Dunedin City Council. Many voluntary, statutory and other agencies are involved in the Action group, co-operation is the key to the group's success.

Healthy City: Christchurch

Healthy Cities in Christchurch is alive and flourishing. In October 1989, a seminar was held to raise community awareness of Healthy Cities and launch the Community Diagnosis Booklet, *Health Influencing Factors*. Following the Healthy Cities Seminar people registered their interest in becoming involved in making Christchurch a Healthy City. Further meetings have been held to discuss future direction. Action so far includes the setting up of an interim planning committee to ensure that promotion of the Healthy Cities concept continues. Political support has been given by the Mayor of Christchurch and the Chairman of the Canterbury Area Health Board to the establishment of a Healthy Cities co-ordinator jointly funded by both agencies. Management of both organizations are now pursuing the implementation of the joint venture.

The framework of an Intersectoral Group has been set up and the goal is to establish a social, economic and physical environment supportive of Healthy City action in the city. Activities have continued in Christchurch since John Ashton's visit in 1988 and have included the following:

1 Vision workshops, with various community groups on what a Healthy City is, have been very successful in focusing attention on the concept and for getting ideas for action.
2 Creative action has included a large mural painted by school pupils. Cashmere High School students wrote and presented their own Healthy Christchurch play and this was incorporated into a national television programme that carried an item on Healthy Cities.
3 Logos were prepared by members of a community-based work scheme for unemployed young people; one was selected for the Christchurch project.
4 A video has been produced outlining the key health issues facing Christchurch and how a Healthy Cities approach can help by providing a forum for joint action.

Healthy City: Palmerston North

John Ashton's visit in 1988 was the catalyst for the start of a three-way partnership to develop Palmerston North as a healthy city. The partnership between the Maori *tangata whenua* of the city, the City Council and the Health Development Unit (now part of the Manawatu-Wanganui Area Health Board established in 1989) is a strong foundation for community action. A steering group was established and continued to focus on Healthy City initiatives over 1988 and 1989 with the help of a full time co-ordinator.

The Area Health Board and Council formally endorsed the project and both staff and elected members became actively involved. Initially there was resistance to yet another committee in the city and it became crucial to reassure community groups and agencies that the Healthy Cities group was a forum for sharing and networking across sectors, not for duplicating what others were doing.

The Steering Group set out both to create debate about what a Healthy City is especially in schools and to acknowledge the numerous models of good practice within the city. Personnel changes within the group and the restructuring of most city sectors saw the group lose impetus. Personnel changes especially involving key managers in sectors and elected representatives mean that Healthy City groups must have a long-term strategy for development: this has been Palmerston North's biggest lesson.

Another co-ordinator has been appointed and the group is focusing on environmental projects within the city timed to coincide with the 1990 World Health Day theme of 'Our Planet: Our Health, Think Globally: Act Locally'. A recycling pilot scheme involving two city streets and some thirty households will provide a focus for the Healthy City initiative. The scheme aims to raise awareness of waste management issues, to involve residents in collective action and to create a ground swell of interest for wider community environmental action by using the scheme as a model of good practice. Support for the scheme has come from the Regional and City Councils, from staff and students at Massay University and the Area Health Board.

Healthy City strategies of vision workshops, acknowledging models of good practice and developing health status reports on communities are being interwoven into the approach that the Area Health Board is evolving with the communities it serves.

Conclusion

Healthy Cities provides us in New Zealand with both an opportunity and a challenge. An opportunity to become an active member of our global village by acting locally in our communities, towns, cities and on the world stage for our country to lead by example within the Pacific and beyond. The challenge is to overcome the apathy that geographical isolation and our environmentally rich country encourages us to develop. Mother Earth is a complex organism.

He wahine, he whenua, i ngaro ai te tangata.

Woman and land are the same, without them people will not survive.

It is up to us. By working together we will make the difference between existing and living.

Acknowledgements

The authors wish to thank Margaret Devlin, Jo Herbert, Louise Croot, Robyn Judge, Jan Maulder and Norma Livingstone.

References

Ashton, J. and Seymour, H. (1988) *The New Public Health*, Milton Keynes: Open University Press.

Davey, J.A. (1987) *Social Policy Options*, Planning Council PO Box 5066, Wellington, New Zealand.

Department of Statistics (1990) *Monthly Unemployment Statistics*. Wellington: Department of Statistics, February.

Franklin, S.H. (1978) *Trade, Growth and Anxiety*, Wellington, New Zealand: Methuen.

Gawenda, M. (1989) 'Going it Alone', *Time* 1 May: 10–22.

Lower Hutt City Council (1988) Unpublished minutes of a meeting in December, Wellington, New Zealand: Lower Hutt City Council.

Minister of Health (1989) *A New Relationship*, Kit including New Zealand Health Charter, New Zealand Health Goals and Targets and A Contract for Area Health Boards, available from Department of Health PO Box 5013 Wellington, New Zealand.

Naisbett, J. (1984) *Megatrends: Ten Directions Transforming Our Lives*, London: Future Macdonald.

Sharing Control: A policy Study of Responsiveness and Devolution in the Statutory Social Services (1988) Wellington, New Zealand: Government Printer.

WHO (World Health Organisation) (1978) *Alma Ata 1977 Primary Health Care*, Geneva: WHO/UNICEF.

WHO, Health and Welfare Canada, Canadian Public Health Association (1986) *Ottawa Charter for Health Promotion*, Coperhagen: WHO.

23

Canberra

Antoinette Ackermann and Judy Whyte

Introduction

Many Canberrans have been involved in the establishment of the Healthy Cities Project. This pilot project occurred during an interesting period in the life of our city with the advent of self-government early in 1989. The involvement of members of the community, senior administrators and local politicians has been an important factor in the development of Healthy Cities Canberra and their continuing commitment encourages the momentum established over the three years. Our achievements were many, not the least being the personal development of those closely involved, and we are pleased to share our story with other cities and communities.

The project's work during these three years was focused at two levels of community development. First, people were encouraged to participate in community and health programmes in the city. Second, co-operation between decision-makers about policies affecting the well-being of the community was encouraged across a wide range of interests. These included education, town planning, environmental conservation, the media and so on. Issues raised during the three years of Healthy Cities Canberra include the difficulties in implementing the Healthy Cities concept within city management *and* the community, defining community and high expectations for change. The following account is based on a series of planning, progress and evaluation reports developed during the three-year pilot project. The authors were involved as Co-ordinator and as a community member involved through various committees and working groups.

The city

Canberra as a planned city and Australia's National Capital has many features which are particular to its situation. The Australian Capital Territory (ACT) was created in 1911 to house the Australian Federal Parliament and the Commonwealth Public Service in a city to be named 'Canberra', an Aboriginal word meaning 'meeting place'. The Federal Government controlled and administered the ACT through a federal minister and department until the advent of self-government in 1989.

The ACT is located in south-eastern New South Wales and has a population of 273,000. Canberra, the metropolitan area, occupies 208 of the 2,400 square metres and is built on land used for grazing sheep prior to the city and suburban development. The building of national offices, service and residential areas began slowly with a major period of growth from the 1950s. Early planning emphasized metropolitan development from the main civic and central area through a series of new towns within the valley systems which preserved hills and ridges in their natural state. These park and garden areas together with a series of artificial lakes provide for a large outdoor recreation area with 4 hectares per 1,000 inhabitants. Towns are linked through an arterial road system with divisions into neighbourhoods each capable of supporting a primary school, shopping centre and community facilities. The national buildings and the areas around them are seen as important to all Australians, so their planning and administration is retained by our Federal Government.

The early development of the city had depended on migration, often compulsory for public servants, from other cities. During the 1980s there was a slowing down in annual growth of the population, with less migration. The higher than average percentage of young adults and families is slowly being balanced with an increase in those over 60 years of age who now make up 9 per cent of the population.

The Canberra community is relatively affluent because the middle-range income is higher than the national average. This has resulted in a greater than normal 'rich–poor' gap for those on lower incomes. Government housing and subsidized housing have been a feature of the development of Canberra and, at present, there is a large range of housing available for the disadvantaged and a number of community-based refuges. Some people claim that there is very little, if any, substandard housing, however, for others there is a sense of the 'hidden poor' in this green and clean city.

Over half the ACT work-force is employed in the public service with a large percentage of the other workers involved in servicing this 'industry'. This has resulted in a population with higher levels of formal education than in other states and a limited range of career opportunities. There are obvious implications for Canberra's young people. They stay at school longer than those in other states with more going on to tertiary education.

Canberra's role as National Capital has led to 'boom and bust' cycles as the amount of money available to the ACT alters with changes in government policy. The rapid growth of new suburbs has caused problems of isolation, transport difficulties and problems in the provision of local and neighbourhood shops and services.

Comments across the nation about 'Canberra', and what 'Canberra' does most frequently refer to the Federal Government and the 'fat cats' who govern the country, so that the identity of the city for its inhabitants is often ignored. For those of us who live here this is a continual conflict for the image of our city. So, applying the Healthy Cities concept to Canberra was a challenge in many ways, not the least its organization and ownership in a planned city where the public service dominates.

Healthy Cities Canberra: the project

From the beginning those involved wanted to find a way to base Healthy Cities Canberra firmly in the community. At the same time we needed support and commitment from the bureaucrats or decision-makers in order to address a wide range of policies and services. Community projects reflecting current and projected social needs of the population were initiated. Working groups of interested citizens guided these projects. Workshops and meetings were held to encourage policies for positive well-being. In late 1987 an intersectoral steering committee was established with representatives from town planning, the arts, community and health services, media, education, social services, trades and labour, private industry, migrant and ethnic communities, medicine, city management and community health.

The struggle to achieve the participation of both the community and the people in powerful positions, that is the bottom-up and top-down approach, is reflected in the process of administration as the project developed. During the pilot project from late 1986 to early 1990, Healthy Cities Canberra's phases of development included a pre-pilot phase, an establishment and review phase, a consolidation phase and a transition phase. In establishing Healthy Cities in Canberra, much time was spent in the early days consulting with key people and organizations gaining support and involvement for this ecological approach to promoting well-being. As time went on, political as well as social considerations dictated the direction of the project. Thus, constant review and assessment of how a Healthy Cities approach could work positively for the people of Canberra was necessary.

Visions

Visions for a Healthy City: Canberra

On a number of occasions the Vision Workshop format was used to establish contact with groups and individuals, to assist their understanding and involve them in the project, and to develop a focus for action. A total of fourteen

Vision Workshops were held involving approximately 400 individuals. Participants came from a wide range of community and professional areas. According to these citizens, 'A Healthy Canberra is . . .' a city which focuses its attention on seven major areas:

1 nutrition
2 a clean environment
3 social and financial equity
4 good community interaction (co-operation and support networks)
5 accessible public transport
6 recreation facilities (parks, festivals, outdoor activities)
7 neighbourhood security.

These areas were seen overwhelmingly as being the responsibility of public policy-makers particularly in areas such as the environment, economics, employment, education, food, industry, transport, and housing. Although the traditional areas of health, that is health education and medical care, were identified they did not carry the weight of these other areas. This particular balance between allocation of responsibilities may be unique to Canberrans who see themselves as citizens of a 'planned' city. It raises questions about the early and continuing participation of members of the community in the planning and development of new towns and cities.

Visions for a future Healthy Cities Programme in Canberra

In January 1989 the Health and Democracy Working Group developed a key document on Community Participation and Consumer Consultation (Janne 1989). This provided a clear statement concerning shared responsibility for genuine consultation between policy-makers and the wider community. In May 1989 the Healthy Cities Canberra staff with the members of the management and evaluation groups met together to review their achievements and make projections for future activities. Again the strategy used was one of visions and projections into the next decade. This group confirmed the increasing emphasis of the project towards activities which inform policy-makers and planners of their potential role in creating a healthier city and in bringing the wider community into the planning process. The outcomes from this workshop were then used as a resource for the design of a strategic plan.

For us, working with visions provided an uplifting and positive approach to planning which the traditional needs analysis with its focus on the problems and negatives of the situation cannot match. This futures or visions planning format was basic to the overall Healthy Cities Canberra process.

Community participation and co-operation

Over the three years a number of Working Groups met regularly to plan and monitor specific projects. The focus for these groups related to special areas of concern identified through the vision workshops and planning meetings. Groups included

1 Health and Democracy Consultative Group
2 Meeting Places Working Group
3 Healthy Cities, Healthy Schools Working Group
4 Youth and Alcohol Task Group
5 Food and Tucker Working Group
6 Healthy Health Care in Hospitals Working Group
7 Environment Forum Working Group
8 Evaluation Group.

Forty-five working group members represented a range of interest areas in public and private sectors. A total of 106 agencies collaborated in the community projects, 38 of which were government based, the remaining 68 being non-government organizations.

Community projects as examples of good practice emerged from or became the focus for the Groups. All projects were clearly based on the New Public Health principles. There was a particular emphasis on collaboration and co-operation with the various interest groups and individuals already involved in specific issues or working in a particular area. Key individuals and representatives from the interest groups became core members of the Working Groups or acted as 'friends'. This provided support and a structure through which Healthy Cities Canberra community-based activities could be extended.

During the first year of the pilot study it was important to establish projects which could demonstrate the value of a comprehensive approach to promoting equitable public health. The aim was to initiate and encourage community initiatives which reflected healthy social and physical environments, community participation and action, individual empowerment through advocacy and mediation strategies, and reorientation of resources towards health promotion in all community services. Table 23.1 provides a 'snapshot' of the Working Groups, their major aim, and projects successfully completed during the pilot study.

Two case studies drawn from the three-year pilot project are summarized below. The 'Open Day on the Common' and 'Schools are for Living in!' projects reflect how individuals, community groups and public administration contribute to developing community participation and healthy public policy in action.

Open Day on the Common

The major focus of the Meeting Places Working Group during the early months of 1989 was a community participation and development programme on the south side of Canberra – Open Day on Narrabundah Common.

The aim of the Open Day was to enhance the well-being of a local community by providing a supportive community environment in which people

Table 23.1 Working group according to aim and completed projects

Working group	Aim	Completed projects
Health and Democracy	To ascertain citizen participation in community planning and ways this may be increased	• Use of community houses: workshop • Youth accommodation consultation • Think Tank Community Consultation and Consumer Participation • Consultation on 'Search Conference' for new Legislative Assembly
Meeting Places	To create accessible meeting places through community involvement	• Social and learning exchange at a local shopping mall • Open Day on the Common: a neighbourhood family day
Healthy Schools, Healthy City	To encourage schools to use a New Public Health framework for planning and review	• Evaluation of Primary School • 'Schools are for living in' Project: schools as places of well-being
Youth and Alcohol	To reduce the amount of alcohol abuse amongst young people	• TV advertisements designed and co-ordinated by young people • Non-alcohol drinks recipes designed and co-ordinated by young people as mature alternative to alcohol
Food and Tucker	To promote better nutritional status for older people, unemployed adults and those at risk of cardiovascular disease	• 'Dentures for Pensioners' Project reduced backlog in waiting list for denture repair
Healthy Health Care	To enhance non-technical aspects of patient care in hospitals	• Consultation and Work-in-Hospitals with selected local hospital unit
Environment Forum	To promote collaboration amongst environment groups and individuals	• Environment forum with initiation and support for environment activities
Evaluation	To evaluate the Healthy Cities Canberra	• Evaluation report of Healthy Cities Canberra Pilot Project • Representation on National Evaluation Subcommittee

could actively participate, and share in promoting a sense of identity with their local community. An inter-agency planning group met monthly to plan the day. Agencies included Southside Community Services, Narrabundah Health Centre, Narrabundah Tertiary and Further Education Outreach, Narrabundah Early Childhood Education Centre and the Heraldry and Genealogy Society. Other community and service organizations participating on the Day included Dairy Farmers Milk Co-operative, Canberra Building Society, CIG Gas (for the balloons), Raja Yoga, Brindabella Community Arts Association, Narrabundah Salvation Army Band and the Canberra City Band. Healthy Cities Canberra played a co-ordinating and facilitating role. Four of the agencies share a piece of common land, hence the title of the project.

Activities included displays and information by the participating agencies, children's activities, a meditation and peace tent, community art and music performances, ACT Fire Brigade and Police Rescue demonstrations, free milk and fruit juice, free balloons and an art and craft exhibition. A Graffiti Wall and Wishing Well provided opportunities for local residents to comment on or make a wish for their community – a kind of visions for the future activity.

An estimated 300 people from the local neighbourhood attended the event which attracted broad media coverage. Open Day on the Common was well supported by government, non-government and voluntary organizations. It is planned that the Open Day will be a continuing event in this neighbourhood.

Schools are for Living in!

This project was initiated by the Healthy Schools, Healthy City Working Group and received the full support of the local Department of Education and was funded and endorsed by the Canberra office of IBM (Computers) Australia Ltd. IBM made a grant for administrative and publicity costs as well as providing two computers for schools entering the most outstanding projects at primary and secondary levels.

The aim of the project was to create healthier, more pleasant schools, and encourage greater involvement with the wider school community. To participate, students and staff at a number of pre-school, primary and secondary schools were to develop projects which demonstrated ways in which their school was creating a supportive environment, strengthening community participation and action, developing individual skills, and orientating school facilities and services towards the pursuit of good health.

In making awards for the most outstanding projects, the selection panel were looking for plans which demonstrated:

1 the physical and social aspects of school life which are conducive to good health
2 a creative approach to whatever issue the school chose to work on
3 evidence of change in some aspects of the school at the conclusion of the project

4 evidence of continuing plans for the school, based on experience gained from participation in the project
5 evidence of liaison or involvement with the community in which the school is located.

The project was conducted over a nine-month period during 1989. All entrants who successfully participated received a Certificate of Achievement at a special presentation by the Minister for Education. This style of project was perceived as a pilot initiative by the Department of Education. Senior executives in the department are now assessing the impact of the project with a view to developing a more substantial programme for the future.

Hall Primary School provide an example of the style of projects undertaken. Hall is a small village community which has grown up outside the metropolitan area. Hall Primary School's objectives were to develop an awareness of the need for individuals, families, schools and communities to save resources by recycling; to set up at the school, a community recycling centre for Hall Village and surrounding district; to improve the children's knowledge of the value of trees to the environment; to initiate a programme of tree growing and planting for the Hall School students' homes, the Hall Village, surrounding farms and the nearby Yass River Valley, and to develop a pride in the general appearance of Hall Primary School and its immediate grounds.

All the above objectives were fulfilled, and the project continues as a focus for the local community with participation and involvement by many local community organizations and individuals.

City planning through policies for positive health

Healthy Cities Canberra addressed the collaborative healthy public policy approach to city planning in a number of ways. These were:

1 influence on planning through individual constituent members of the Council of Reference (formerly the steering committee) on planning in their sector, e.g. Parks and Conservation Service activities such as lake protection and tree planting, Ethnic Communities Council promotion of cultural links and individual skills together with Arts Council
2 influence on policy-makers in ACT administration through half-day seminars on implementing healthy public policy
3 discussions and dissemination of information on Healthy Cities Canberra and the New Public Health to all political candidates prior to the ACT Government elections
4 involvement of ACT government ministers in activities of the project
5 involvement of other agencies such as media e.g. production of five short videos by Capital 10 TV depicting images of the Healthy Cities approach to better health in Canberra.

Reflections on the pilot project

Influencing forces in the city

Over the three years of the project we can identify a number of forces at work in Canberra. While some of these contributed to smooth progress in Healthy Cities Canberra, others acted as inhibiting forces. They include:

1 physical and environmental factors, e.g. inner city parking, controversy over fluoridated water, planning for a new town centre
2 political events, e.g. the growth of resident action groups, cancellation of community boards by a Federal Minister, frequent changeover of Federal Ministers with ACT responsibilities, arrival of self-government
3 local administration forces, e.g. existence of a senior interdepartmental executive committee, endless restructuring of key agencies managing Canberra (the government sector responsible for health had five name changes in the 1980s)
4 private sector factors, e.g. growth of the private sector share of the economy, a Very Fast Train proposal linking Sydney, Canberra and Melbourne, and a proposal for a Casino
5 *Zeitgeist* (mood of the times) factors, e.g. increase in general environmental awareness, increase in violence, increasing power of anti-smoking lobby, fluctuating economic situation.

An analysis of these factors over the life of Healthy Cities Canberra showed most of the inhibiting forces to be located in the local administrative areas.

Key informant survey

An independent evaluator using a series of interviews undertaken in June and July 1989 elicited the opinions of the majority of seventy key individuals who had had direct contact or involvement in Healthy Cities Canberra. The evaluation was intended to obtain honest opinion from a large and representative sample of Canberrans. These individuals perceived major strengths to be in the vision and concept of the Healthy Cities movement itself, the community development work and the work of those closely involved as a model of good practice. Although there were many positive outcomes the general view appeared to be critical. This was especially so in relation to inadequate funding and support, the low profile, apparently unclear goals and objectives, professional resistance and scepticism at the top.

A strong impression gained by the interviewer was that, despite the general goodwill towards Healthy Cities Canberra and indeed, the areas of strong commitment, the majority of informants were still waiting for Healthy Cities Canberra to amaze them.

Trends and continuing activities

A number of continuing activities can be identified in the city which demonstrate the Healthy Cities concept. Some which continue at the time of writing are Parks and Conservation programmes, 'Milk in Glass' and other recycling programmes, a three-year project aiming to enhance the quality of life of the increasing numbers of older citizens and public advertising of Canberra as a healthy city.

1 The Parks and Conservation sector of the city administration has a clear orientation to the community through its services and its consultative practices. Examples are seen in the community tree-planting days, the development of nature trails, and the organization of community walks including special activities for those with disabilities. Regular consultation with the community occurs through local meetings, questionnaires and informal discussion with both individuals and specific community groups.

2 The ACT Milk Authority with the support of Healthy Cities Canberra is promoting the sale of milk in glass as an environmentally sound alternative to milk in plasticized cardboard cartons and large plastic containers. The citizens of Canberra have responded positively to this and to other re-cycling initiatives.

3 The University of Canberra has established a recycling process, beginning with paper and expanding to other materials. A committee with a range of representatives from across the campus initiates and supports the activities. It organizes an annual environment awareness week and is currently working on a recycling policy to be submitted to the University Council for ratification.

4 A new initiative with a national funding base has a major focus on the social isolation of elderly people. It involves an intersectoral committee and draws on the community structures and processes established by Healthy Cities Canberra.

5 The local media are showing increasing support for the notion of Canberra as a healthy city. A local commercial TV channel with the aid of members of the community, developed a number of short messages illustrating ways towards a healthier city. Themes for the messages were drawn from Vision Workshops conducted through Healthy Cities Canberra in the city centre and parks.

Discussion and conclusion

In Canberra at the end of the pilot phase the big issues for the future are the physical location, funding, and role of Healthy Cities Canberra once this pilot phase is finished. The key individuals surveyed had many instructive comments to make. The overwhelming wish was that Healthy Cities Canberra should continue. The biggest issue was whether the project should be based within the umbrella of a community agency or within an area involved in city administration. It was clear that funding would be needed for some time to come. However, there were fears that Healthy Cities Canberra would get lost in the bureaucracy as well as clear appreciation of the need for a strong community base. There was also recognition that input at both community agency and bureaucratic levels was necessary for Healthy Cities Canberra to achieve its aims. It was also apparent that the private sector, a growing force in the city, needed to be drawn in, in a meaningful and co-operative manner.

It was evident to the key members of the Healthy Cities Canberra network that community projects are its important public face. The vital task at present is to get the five principles of the New Public Health on to the policy and planning agendas of all the ACT agencies so that they can implement decisions using their own skills and resources. The Healthy Cities Canberra Strategic Plan provides specific guidelines as to how this should happen. The Plan also contains practical plans for integrating social justice strategies into programmes and involving the community via private industry sponsorship, educational institutions, the media, arts organisations, youth groups, migrant groups and professional organizations. Individuals will be involved through community health initiatives.

Healthy Cities concepts are to some extent embedded in the life of the city of Canberra. More time is needed to consolidate this, particularly in the light not only of a new self-government structure but also a changed government after an initial six-month period.

Finally there are some aspects of the Healthy Cities Canberra learning process which we feel should be highlighted so that other cities may compare and contrast their own experience with our story. Lessons we have learned to date are as follows:

1 There is pressure to implement the project at all levels, a stressful process if there is inadequate support.
2 There is a problem in trying to engage in this social engineering process with fewer resources than necessary.
3 The Healthy Cities approach arouses high expectations yet the changes hoped for are large scale, and inevitably long term, slow, and show results gradually.
4 The wish to 'give away' skills and resources to others and to 'let go' in project work is a problem for a Healthy Cities team which has a wide-ranging client group – the citizens of their city.
5 There is a need to work through local government structures and initiatives.
6 There is a need to clarify the relationship between community and bureaucratic components of the city – who is 'the Community'?
7 The physical location of Healthy Cities Canberra can bring repercussions which are both positive and negative, i.e. the cottage in a suburban community setting, or a higher profile shopfront setting.
8 Documenting the process raises many issues, including sorting through guidelines for an appropriate brief and making reports relevant to all those involved.

In conclusion, Healthy Cities in Canberra is an important learning process for us all – compulsive, rewarding, sometimes frustrating, occasionally surprising, and always time consuming. Looking back over the three years it is obvious that it is the process of being involved which is a Healthy Cities strength in the longer term.

We appreciate the ever-increasing network of Healthy Cities globally. The encouragement and support from other cities participating in the Healthy Cities movement both in Australia and elsewhere is playing an important role in our development.

Appendix: pilot project phases

Pre-pilot phase

During the pre-pilot phase a working group of bureaucrats with the support of community members and the ACT Community Health Association (ACTCHA) received commitment from the then-named ACT Health Authority and other major ACT agencies. The Health Authority also sponsored the first National Workshop in January 1987 which brought together the three cities proposed for the Healthy Cities Australia. Canberra as a venue for this first Workshop was a logical choice in its role as seat of the Federal Government, given that funding was still being sought.

Establishment phase

The establishment phase saw the appointment of the Co-ordinator, the establishment of an intersectoral Steering Committee, the identification of focus areas through a series of vision workshops and the establishment of working groups for small projects. This included the establishment of an evaluation group. In this phase funding was directed through the Health Authority which provided considerable assistance in the form of accommodation, and administrative and clerical support. An important arrangement during this phase was the establishment of an office in a community house in the older suburb of Ainslie. A review of progress and management structure after almost one year enabled the consolidation of this early work to begin in earnest.

Consolidation phase

The consolidation phase began under a change of financial management with a community group, the ACTCHA, handling funds and the continuing commitment of the Health Authority with important resource support. A new management structure was put in place with a sixteen-member Council of Reference representing an increased range of sectors responsible for direction and policy status and a Management Committee responsible for the day to day management of the project. This new structure assisted in placing Healthy Cities Canberra more effectively in the community. A review of progress at this stage together with the development of a strategic plan provided guidelines for building on to the pilot phase.

Transition phase

A transition phase during the final few months of Federal funding is expected to ensure the establishment of the Healthy Cities concept in the administration and life of the city. During this period a particular focus is on achieving support and commitment equally from the public, private and community sectors as a co-operative venture.

Reference

Janne, G. (1989) *Community Consultation and Consumer Participation Policy Proposal*, Canberra: Healthy Cities Canberra.

24

Noarlunga

Frances Baum and Ann Skewes

Noarlunga is on the southern edge of Adelaide, capital of South Australia –
the driest State in the driest continent. The State is known for its world-class
wine, the biannual Festival of Arts, the Grand Prix and its progressive liberal
tradition that still exerts a strong influence on the State's direction and atmosphere. Adelaide is seen by the rest of Australia as a somewhat effete place
that doesn't live up to the Ocker image celebrated in the louder, brassier
eastern states. Since 1973 the State has been governed by Labour administrations apart from a short period of Liberal government in the early 1980s.

It is hard to describe Noarlunga to those who haven't visited Australia.
It is wedged between the urban sprawl of Adelaide from the north, some of
the best vineyards in Australia to the east and south, with spectacular coastal
areas of long, sandy beaches interspersed by dramatic red cliffs to the west.
The city currently has a population of approximately 75,000, which is projected to grow to over 120,000 by the year 2000 (Dept Environment and
Planning 1985). Typical of many other communities on the outskirts of
major Australian cities, it is home mortgage territory with a high proportion
of families with children: one-third of the population is under 15. Public
health problems include those of inequalities in health status between men
and women and between people in different income groups; stress-related
problems resulting from over-commitment to consumer credit; social isolation, particularly for women, which is aggravated by inflexible and insufficient public transport; environmental problems such as lack of trees and
pollution of the river estuary and beaches.

Europeans visiting Noarlunga, however, would not be struck by problems
but by the wide open spaces, apparently clean air and the ease of living in the
'lucky country'. A recent visitor to Australia from the European office of the
World Health Organization commented that 'the living conditions in many

Australian cities would seem quite marvellous to the inhabitants of cities like Glasgow, Liverpool or Belfast'. But all that is relative and the locals can and do identify health problems.

Like most Healthy Cities Projects the Noarlunga one did not start in a vacuum. It was preceded by community discussion about its health needs in a process leading up to the State Government's decision to build a regional 'Health Village' to be followed by a hospital a few years later. The charter of the Health Village was, in common with other community health centres in South Australia, to develop health promotion initiatives and provide multi-disciplinary primary health care services throughout the Noarlunga area. Part of the planning for the 'Village' included an extensive assessment of community health needs, the results of which were published in a booklet entitled *Noarlunga's Health – Apathy or Action?* (Southern Community Health Research Unit 1985), 2,500 copies of which were distributed to local community groups for discussion and debate (see Plate 24.1).

Local community services have been meeting monthly at a Community Services Forum since the late 1970s and the local Council has considerably strengthened its community services department in response to the increasing urbanization of the area. The ideas from the World Health Organization European Project found fertile ground in Noarlunga and staff at the Health Village saw the opportunity to develop further a community-based approach to health promotion. They joined together with the two other pilot Australian Healthy Cities (Canberra and Illawarra) and were successful in obtaining Federal Government funding which provided for a local project manager and clerical support. The funding was given for a three-year period to pilot the European Healthy Cities approach under Australian conditions.

Like most Healthy Cities projects, the Noarlunga initiative has operated at different levels and used a variety of strategies. In essence these reflect the Ottawa Charter of Health Promotion (WHO *et al.* 1986) on which the Healthy Cities approach is based. Effort is invested in: encouraging more co-operation between local services and agencies; promoting the idea that safeguarding and improving health is the province of a wide range of sectors in the community (for example, education, welfare, housing and recreation); supporting community initiatives aimed at improving the quality of life and the natural environment; encouraging local communities to take action to improve health and defining a vision of what an ideally healthy future Noarlunga might look like. Healthy Cities is then, working with two basic strategies of bringing about change: a 'top-down' model that concentrates on working with the local and State government departments in the way described above and along side this a 'bottom-up' approach that is driven by local people who are not employed in government agencies and who define issues of importance and work alongside government employees in achieving their goals. Inevitably there has been some tension between these two strategies. Community members have felt frustrated by the relative slow pace at which the more technocratic model brings about change, feeling it should be more responsive to their concerns, while some of the government officials

NOARLUNGA'S HEALTH
– Apathy or Action ?

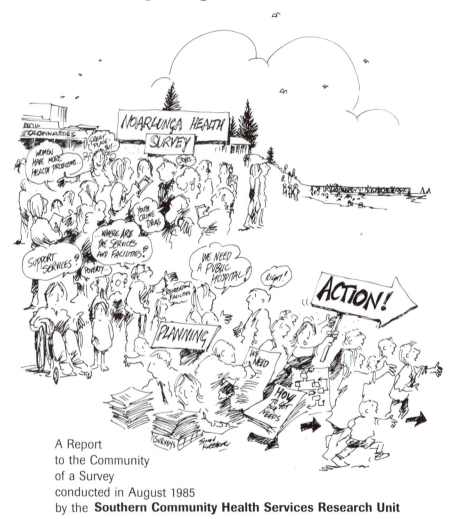

A Report
to the Community
of a Survey
conducted in August 1985
by the **Southern Community Health Services Research Unit**

Figure 24.1   Front cover of the booklet entitled *Noarlunga's Health – Apathy or Action?*

may find it hard to cope with the less bureaucratic methods and objectives of the community members. How these tensions work out in the future remains to be seen. The Noarlunga experience does suggest that Healthy Cities provides a mechanism for dealing with the inevitable conflicts that arise from the tensions between the different sectors and approaches involved.

The Healthy Cities Project is housed and administered in the Health Village which is based at a large regional centre with shops, government offices and transport services to Adelaide. This Health Village was heralded as an innovative approach to the provision of primary health care when it was opened in 1985. Its policy statement puts emphasis on a social health approach with a strong health promotion focus. Programmes include primary medical care and a range of other health services (speech pathology (speech therapy), physiotherapy, psychology, social work). Strategies range from one-to-one service delivery to community development approaches. Healthy Cities has then been based in an organization that had similiar objectives to those of the project. This has obvious benefits. The one drawback has been that some of the existing health workers have perceived duplication of their work with that of the Healthy Cities Project. Resolving this has been one of the challenges for the project as it has evolved. The project is managed by a committee which meets monthly and contains representatives from government departments and four community members. All members have a high commitment to the project and its aims. A Reference Committee has also been established. The project has received formal endorsement from the South Australian Government and the Noarlunga City Council. This formal endorsement has been followed by impressive commitment to the project by local politicians, all of whom have been willing to endorse the project by attending public meetings, offering letters of support, and by recognizing the work of the project in their speeches.

One of the challenges the Healthy Cities Project has faced in Noarlunga has been that, unlike most European cities which are governed by two layers of administration (National and City Government), in most Australian communities there are three (Federal, State and Local). This has complicated the task of co-ordinating services. It has also highlighted tensions between the different tiers of government, particularly between Local Government and larger 'resource rich' Federal and State Authorities.

A supportive and active cadre of community members have worked closely with salaried workers on a variety of projects. This type of contribution is typified by one of the community representatives on the Management Committee. She is the co-ordinator of a pressure group established to address the problem of pollution in the local river estuary. The group has highlighted a reluctance by State and local authorities to assume responsibility for cleaning up the river to render it safe for recreational use. Healthy Cities plays a facilitating role in projects such as this by supporting the pressure group with advice, resources and lobbying. Its work has led to extensive media coverage and prompted the State Minister of Environment, Planning and Water Resources to set up a Task Force to study the problem. This Task Force is recommending ways in which the river can be cleaned up. Plans have also been made to make the river estuary a recreation park and hand its management over to the National Parks and Wildlife Services. A similar group was established a couple of years ago to campaign for better water quality in the Noarlunga area (the outer southern suburbs of Adelaide have experienced poorer water quality than the rest of the city, where the low quality of water is, in any case, legendary). This group was successful in having all its demands met by the end of 1988. Group members were enthusiastic in attributing part of their success to the support they received from the Healthy Cities project. Other projects with strong community backing and supported by Healthy Cities have been: a campaign for a formal community park, a school-based education programme, community awareness of the needs of carers of elderly and disabled people; action to improve the provision of public transport in the area; obtaining funding for a master plan to re-green the southern area of Adelaide; and support to a group developing a suburban farm. The Healthy Cities Project, along with the spirit of the times, has been greened over its three years of existence. This greening has been driven by a community interest and concern with the varied environmental projects. One initiative which aims to foster a co-ordinated approach to environmental health issues is the development of an Environmental Health Management Plan for Noarlunga. As an equivalent to a city health plan this encompasses a range of aspects, from housing and hazardous chemicals to paper recycling and air quality. But the attention was not just on the problems. It was also on the desirable features of Noarlunga (such as the beaches and open spaces) which the community wanted preserved and enhanced. So through workshops and surveys of schools and community groups, priority issues were identified and research undertaken. One interesting outcome was the creation of a number of new positions for Health Surveyors (environmental health officers) at the Council. Another was the partnerships and alliances which were formed. For example, the local environmental watchdog group working side by side with government bodies, a significant change from their previously polarized positions and the essence of Healthy Cities in action.

Another of the undoubted successes of the project has been the monthly magazine, *Health Works* (see Figure 24.2). Over six hundred copies are distributed to community groups and schools; it provides a forum for the reporting of local health issues, announcing future events and programmes and placing an emphasis on activities that promote health which are taking place in various places in the community.

Perhaps the most successful community venture has been the 'visions of a Healthy Noarlunga project', which culminated in the birth of the 'Dream Machine'. This started with a series of workshops with community members to define their vision of Noarlunga as a future Healthy City. These workshops were modelled on those developed in Toronto, Canada. Using guided imagery they encouraged participants (approximately 300 from community groups ranging from the local Rotary Club to kindergartens) to identify elements of their ideally healthy Noarlunga. These visions were then used by a community artist (funded by Foundation South Australia which was established by the State Government and financed by moneys from tobacco taxation, to sponsor sporting, artist and health promotion initiatives) to develop these ideas, in consultation with community groups and other artists to produce the 'Dream Machine'. This highly colourful, inventive and attrac-

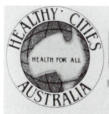

Health Works

NEWSLETTER OF HEALTHY CITIES : NOARLUNGA

Healthy Cities concept launched

Over 200 local and interstate guests packed the auditorium at Noarlunga Health Services on Sunday 28th June, to witness Dr. Neal Blewett officially launch the exciting "Healthy Cities — Australia" Project

The Launch commenced with community artists, Simon Kneebone and Tony King creating murals depicting images of health in the community, as put forward by members of the audience.

The Mayor of Noarlunga, Mr. Ray Gilbert stated that "the Healthy Cities concept was only a small step, nevertheless a significant one" and that the Noarlunga Council "was pleased to be involved as an active partner in "Healthy Cities: Noarlunga", and a contributor to "Healthy Cities — Australia"

Professor Dennis Calvert, Chairperson of "Healthy Cities: Illawarra", who has recently returned from a Healthy Cities conference in Dusseldorf, said "the European cities had similar difficulties to Australian Cities, although a different balance. We can learn from the rest of the world, but the rest of the world has a lot to learn from us."

Dr. John Cornwall then introduced the Hon. Neal Blewett and offered enthusiastic support to the Healthy Cities concept.

Dr. Blewett stated he "had a conviction that Health Departments are not just for curing the ill", and supported this by describing the new priorities in the Commonwealth Department of Health.

These changes included increasing health education, furthering education of health professionals to increase expertise, improving pharmaceuticals accessibility, supporting a structural change in industry and local environments aimed at increasing safety, as well as supplying universal health insurance through Medicare.

A major display highlighted the Health Cities Project (for exhibition in public venues around Australia), made an appropriate back-drop to the official launch.

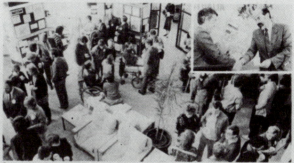

Section of guests present at the Launch. **Insert:** *Handing over of cheque to National President Australian Community Health Association, Richard Hicks*

Healthy Cities Australia
What it will mean to Noarlunga

One of the central aims of the Noarlunga Healthy Cities Project will be to develop co-operation and commitment from other government departments (like education, welfare, transport etc.) and community services not traditionally involved in the health sector or concerned about health issues

The intention is to build on a survey conducted by the Southern Community Health Services Research Unit, which demonstrated clear social patterns of health and illness in Noarlunga. This survey highlighted areas such as transport, housing, employment, income level and social supports as having a significant impact on people's health. The Healthy Cities Project will work towards making Noarlunga a healthier place to live by linking appropriate authorities and agencies together in a co-ordinated approach to health promotion.

Noarlunga played an important role in the launch of the Healthy Cities Australia Project in June, and in July in hosting a National Healthy Cities Workshop. The workshop, held on 13th and 14th July, supplied an opportunity for local workers and interested members of the public to hear more about Healthy Cities.

In the opening session of the workshop an overview of the Healthy Cities Australia Project was presented with updates from each of the pilot cities.

For further information contact Ann Skewes on 326 0433

The Healthy Cities Project in Noarlunga is being developed by an Interim Steering Committee which includes representatives from Noarlunga Health Services, Southern Community Health Services Research Unit, Southern Womens Health and Community Centre, the Social Health Office, the Health Development Foundation, Noarlunga City Council and the Noarlunga Community Services Forum. The intention is that this committee have broad representation and participation by both public and private agencies in the area and the local community

Welcome

Welcome to the first edition of "Health Works", the Newsletter of "Healthy Cities: Noarlunga". The publication is intended to facilitate the distribution of information between local agencies and community groups with a particular focus in the area of health promotion

"Health Works" will endeavour to disseminate information on programmes and services available in the southern area, highlight issues in the area of health promotion and publicise new campaigns and other promotional activities so, "Health Works" will work best if it incorporates information for you and about you.

Figure 24.2 The Noarlunga Healthy Cities Newsletter.

tive art-piece was launched at a community picnic which attracted considerable local and media interest. It was also the focus of a 'Noarlunga 2000 and Beyond' Community Day. This venture was successful not only because it involved so many people, but also because it involved the hard to reach, especially those who found little of relevance in the Healthy Cities approach. Significant among these was the local Aboriginal group. They found the artwork of the 'Dream Machine' a powerful vehicle through which to express their concepts of life, past, present and future. From this perspective, the value of community arts cannot be overrated. The contribution is significant, both in terms of the product or what is created as well as the process by which it is achieved. What remains in Noarlunga is a challenging community statement about the future.

The initiatives that Healthy Cities Noarlunga has been involved with during just three years of operation have been considerable and have been done with relatively little money. The grant from the Commonwealth Department of Community Services and Health for the pilot amounted to A\$55,000 per city per annum. In the 1988/89 financial year it was estimated that an additional A\$164,950 was gained in terms of staff resources and other assistance to the project from local sources. Evaluation of the project indicates strong support from local service providers for the project's philosophy and approach. The evaluation was designed to provide feedback to the project managers and has highlighted some challenges for Healthy City projects like Noarlunga's. Chief among these is the need for an effective way of involving local communities that is neither tokenistic nor purely for the purpose of gaining endorsement for decisions that have already been taken. Community members involved in Healthy Cities Noarlunga have seen it as a vehicle for gaining access to service-providers and decision-makers in local government. Through Healthy Cities they have a direct line of communication to senior managers in these organizations. Instead of being blocked by bureaucratic processes they become astute and knowledgeable about how to utilize these systems to their best advantage. This process makes them more powerful and so reinforces their position as valid and equal partners in the Healthy Cities strategy. However, this kind of involvement does not come about overnight; Healthy Cities, like other community development projects, has recognized that equal and productive partnerships with community members and paid workers poses problems. Those involved in the project feel that they have made headway in doing this. Consultation has been thorough and reasonably extensive. The admission by the Management Committee, mid-way through the pilot period, that despite the successes there was still room for improvement meant a major goal for 1989 was the development of a broader base of community input to the project. This was done with the help of initiatives such as the Dream Machine Project described above.

A further challenge has been to convince the sceptics. The ideas embodied in the Healthy Cities Project are innovative and seem to appeal most to those who thrive on lateral thinking. In fact the Healthy Cities Project is best conceived not as a project (which implies something static and fixed) but rather as an approach which is flexible, fluid and welcomes adaptation. The central message that the project in Noarlunga has tried to impart to service providers is that they should reassess the way they approach their work, ask themselves whether they could do things differently or more creatively to achieve better and more desirable outcomes for their clients. This type of change also takes time. People may feel threatened, their imaginations may not be captured by the potential of a new approach or they may simply be too busy with their current work. Common statements often made in this regard are 'it's too hard', 'it's not tangible', 'it's not proven'. In Noarlunga the project is slowly winning over key stake-holders. Indeed, part of the strategy has been educative: talks to a wide variety of local community groups, presentations to the local council, school principals, the executive of the State Health Commission, the local teaching hospital and numerous conference presentations. While the philosophies behind Healthy Cities do not have universal appeal these presentations are usually received enthusiastically. There are, of course, still sceptics who prefer not to be challenged into new ways of approaching their work. One sign of the project's success will be the time when some of the sceptics change their way of operating and do not attribute this to Healthy Cities. This is the way of all good community development exercises.

Moving the project from a pilot exercise, funded by the Federal Government to a continuing initiative with local backing is the final challenge. As a pilot project, considerable emphasis was on results; 'getting the runs on the board' and 'doing lots with little'. To some extent this was at the cost of building the coalitions and alliances necessary to secure the longevity of the project and resourcing beyond the pilot phase. Another aspect of this is that the community sometimes sees little value in pilot 'experimental' schemes. They are not there to be experimented upon and accordingly are wary and reluctant to make a commitment to something which is short-lived. This is particularly relevant to Healthy Cities which is dependent on community participation and the considerable investment of individuals. Once began, it cannot be stopped by the stroke of a bureaucratic pen but just what it will look like in the future remains to be seen. Our most optimistic view is that the vision embodied in the Dream Machine becomes the reality of Noarlunga's future!

References

Department of Environment and Planning, Forecasting and Land Monitoring Unit (1985) *Projection of Population by Age and Sex for Local Government Areas in the Adelaide Statistical Division, 1981–2001*, Adelaide: DEP, S.A. Government.
Southern Community Health Research Unit (1985) *Noarlunga's Health – Apathy or Action?*, Adelaide: SCHRU, Southern Australian Health Commission.
WHO (World Health Organisation), Health and Welfare Canada, Canadian Public Health Association (1986) *Ottawa Charter for Health Promotion*, Copenhagen: WHO.